OWN THE
BUMP

'Yoga is the best exercise during pregnancy, as it really stretches the body and calms it down. It teaches you breathing techniques which help you during labour, and somehow prepare your body to accept labour pains that are inevitable. It helps your body from inside out' —Maria Goretti, actor

'My pregnancy was very stressful. I lost my father when I was 4 months' pregnant and right after that, I started working on my election campaign. It was stressful, and I was always on my feet. [During] those tough days, what helped me was yoga. I took time out and joined a class. That was my "me time". I did my stretches and exercises for pregnancy, and [practised] breathing techniques. More than anything else, that one hour relaxed me and my baby as well. I recommend yoga as a must, especially during pregnancy'—Priya Dutt, politician

'I had the best pregnancy. I ate everything in sight, it was my golden ticket to binge every day without feeling super guilty! But a few things that kept me healthy were the things that I learnt from Payal, the breathing exercises, the stretches, etc. My advice for expectant mothers is eat healthy and try and do and enjoy yoga with the consent of your doctor'—Amrita Arora Ladak, actor

'When I was pregnant, I started practising breathing exercises with an instructor who would come to teach my husband. That calmed me down a lot because I am quite a hyper person by nature. Then when I started proper yoga sessions with Payal, I started loving this way of staying fit'—Shaheen Abbas, jewellery designer

'For me yoga has always been a space where I can find a sense of calm. As I faced the challenge of labour and impending motherhood, it helped me clear my mind and focus on the present. Yoga sorted out my aches and pains and helped me remember to breathe, increase my flexibility and strength for childbirth'—Laila Khan, artist

'Yoga is an investment I made in my body about five years ago. You know how they say muscles have muscle memory. In the same way, when your body learns to be flexible and elastic, it knows how to stretch, and I think that helped me a lot when I delivered my twins.

I was bigger than most people, and light yoga helped me a lot with breathing and staying calm. I would recommend yoga to all the women who are planning to start a family. This will help a lot later, when you do conceive and deliver, and it'll make the process a lot more easier'—Teejay Sidhu, actress, film producer and radio jockey

'Payal's yoga is the best thing that happened to me. I didn't do any exercise when I was pregnant, which led to me weighing 85 kg by the end of it and looking like a baby elephant. When I attended a get-together after my deliveries, I hadn't shed much of the weight that I had gained and there were flying comments about how I looked. I realized that I had let go of my routine of staying fit. I started with morning walks. Then I started practising yoga with Payal and her husband Manish. The entire process of learning yoga from them has been very rewarding for me. Apart from being physically fit and agile, my mind is completely at peace. I have been so satisfied that I have even introduced my children to yoga'—Sridevi, actor

PAYAL GIDWANI TIWARI

OWN THE BUMP

A COMPLETE **GUIDE** ON
YOGA FOR PREGNANCY

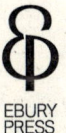

EBURY
PRESS

An imprint of Penguin Random House

EBURY PRESS

USA | Canada | UK | Ireland | Australia
New Zealand | India | South Africa | China | Singapore

Ebury Press is part of the Penguin Random House group of companies
whose addresses can be found at global.penguinrandomhouse.com

Published by Penguin Random House India Pvt. Ltd
4th Floor, Capital Tower 1, MG Road,
Gurugram 122 002, Haryana, India

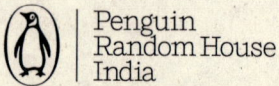

Penguin
Random House
India

First published in Ebury Press by Penguin Random House India 2018

Copyright © Payal Gidwani Tiwari 2018
Foreword copyright © Malaika Arora Khan 2018

ISBN 9780143440208

Typeset in Adobe Garamond Pro by Manipal Digital Systems, Manipal

Printed at Repro India Limited

To Srideviji—you will always remain in our hearts.
We will love you forever.

Contents

Acknowledgements

My first and foremost gratitude is to God, the almighty, the supreme power, for helping me become the medium to reach out to the world. I feel blessed and want to express my thanks to my fans around the world who inspired me to write. The love and affection from my readers made my first book, *From XL to XS*, a national bestseller, selling over 75,000 copies, and encouraged me to write my second book, *Body Goddess*, which won the Raymond Crossword Book Award 2016–17 for the most popular book.

My third book aims to help all mothers-to-be, new mothers as well as couples planning to start a family. Fitness, through all stages of life, should be a priority, and with this book, I want to be able to help everyone enjoy the beautiful change of becoming parents while keeping their fitness in check.

Jacqueline D'Souza has been my right hand through the journey of writing this book, day in, day out. She has managed the commendable feat of juggling it all while holding the fort at our studio Cosmic Fusion, and this book would not have been possible without her. I would also like to thank Ishani Bhattacharya, editorial assistant at Penguin Random House India, who worked with me in giving a complete shape to this book.

I would especially like to thank Ekta Mohanani Kamra for always being there for me. My special thanks to Dr Hemant Brahme, consultant obstetrician and gynaecologist, who took time out from his busy schedule and guided me through every step of this book.

We take traits from the people with whom we spend most of our time. My students taught me patience by bearing with my irregular schedules and giving me their wholehearted support. My family taught me the importance of strength by being by my side through all my ventures. My in-laws made me realize that I can achieve much more than I think I am capable of. My parents are my pillars, for bringing me up and teaching me the invaluable life lessons which have brought me where I am today. The most important person without whom this book and my previous two books would not have been possible is my editor, Milee Ashwarya, editor-in-chief, Penguin Random House India. She has been an integral part of the journey of my books. There are no words grand enough to thank all these bright stars in my life.

My husband, Manish Tiwari, deserves my never-ending gratitude for playing the role of both parents while I wrote this book, standing beside me through thick and thin, and supporting and moulding me in this career. You have always inspired and motivated me to reach great heights in my career.

My son, Sayaan Tiwari, who is my world, who at such a young age understood when I couldn't spend enough time with him or be there for all his activities while I was writing. One day, dear son, you will know why I sat and worked so hard and how this book will help so many people bring young angels just like you, into this world. Thank you, my loving son, for making me a mother and completing my life.

Foreword

To debunk the popular notion that expectant mothers shouldn't exert themselves at all by way of exercise during those nine months, the first step is to realize just how beneficial exercise, particularly yoga, is during this time. As one who has been fit all her life, not exercising during my pregnancy was not an option. After consulting my gynaecologist, I surmised yoga as the way forward for a smoother and less painful delivery.

Since power yoga was out of the question, what with the excessive cardiovascular routines that are an inherent part of this form of yoga, I focused on integral aspects that would not only help during my delivery, but make the preceding nine months a breeze; like deep breathing which would help keep me calm during labour, practising poses that would reverse my shifted sense of body balance and ease my lower back pain. Payal Gidwani Tiwari's set of exercises mentioned in the book address these concerns and provide a possible solution to almost all kinds of problems expecting mothers might face.

The stretches that I practised during my pregnancy were the cat-cow stretch, the warrior pose, the butterfly pose, the mountain pose and the bridge pose. Also, I practised the humming-bee breath and alternate-nostril technique religiously.

The cat-cow, bridge and mountain poses helped in the overall stretching of my spine, easing my acute back pain. They also strengthened my core muscles, making my delivery less painful.

The safe-for-all-trimesters warrior pose was key in improving my body balance and upping my stamina which definitely helped during my labour!

Improving overall flexibility in the pelvic region, the butterfly pose was also a key exercise in alleviating fatigue which permeates the pregnancy months.

And lastly, the breathing techniques I incorporated washed away negative emotions like frustration and distress, keeping me calm at all times.

Regular exercise during your pregnancy is vital, even if it's just a walk or staying active around the house. Remember, as a woman, your body is intrinsically conditioned to carry and nurture another human being, so go forth and stay active; your smooth(er) labour and consequent delivery will be reward enough!

—Malaika Arora Khan, actor

Introduction

Back in the old days, people got married very young and started a family at an early age. Today, the same decisions in life are taken after meticulous planning and weighing of pros and cons by the modern generation. Starting a family in the late teens or early twenties seems incomprehensible, and our grandparents' decisions often seem incredulous, though no less admired.

With the prevalence of the nuclear family structure, both partners are career-oriented with a defined set of goals; they split chores, bills and finances. My husband Manish and I both work and have our roles divided. The responsibilities for our six-year-old son Sayaan are also divided. The upper- and middle-class families today strive to secure their future and build a better home for parenthood. Self-reliant, this generation takes on bigger roles earlier in life and works hard to realize its dreams and aspirations. The desire to start a family comes up only after the couple believes they are in a financially secure and stable stage in their careers. An unplanned pregnancy, in such cases, comes as a surprise.

The lifestyle adaptations an unplanned pregnancy leads to can cause nervousness and worry leading to unaddressed stress between the couple. Having no contingency plan could strain their existing relationship, mentally and physically challenging and pressurizing the couple, leading to drastic decisions at times. It is important to note the increased prevalence of single parenting. Having a good communication and support system in such situations becomes essential for helping the couple sail through this situation without harming their relationship.

Parenthood is an important phase in a couple's relationship, which can be a roller-coaster ride. People coming from various classes face this situation, but not all resort to termination of the pregnancy if it is unplanned. People who are working for a daily wage often work hard to make ends meet and bring up their children, who then grow up to make their parents proud in some way or the other. Let us take the example of Rajan and Savita, a young couple who had recently moved to Delhi from a small town in Uttar Pradesh for better job opportunities. Rajan and Savita soon started working at a call centre. They lived in a rented accommodation which had water and electricity issues. They planned to save up enough to move to a better accommodation after a year or so. Seven months after moving to the big city, Savita realized she was pregnant. After breaking the news to Rajan, they sat down to discuss this change. They didn't have enough money saved up to move to a better place to raise a child and were worried about the health expenses coming up. They decided to talk to their friends and seek advice. Their friends helped them find a better accommodation. The steps they took of sitting down and discussing the change and seeking a support system worked out in their favour. It is always better if you plan and discuss so that stress and other factors do not affect your life. There are cases where couples do not have enough support and then the only difference is that the struggle is greater.

We do remark, often, that the lives and times of our grandparents and parents were much simpler. Living in a joint family, all work and finances were usually divided between men of the household, while most of the women stayed home to attend to domestic chores. They cooked, cleaned and raised children, content and at peace, with minimal extraneous concerns on a different level—only that the family had three square meals and children received a good education. It seems plausible then, that they had so many children before their 30s and did not go through the same stress of trying to provide for their child which a nuclear family set-up often entails. For example, Kanika, a journalist, was living with her joint family during her first pregnancy in Delhi. She appreciated the fact that she had so many people around her during the many changes she went through. She felt the support from her in-laws and relatives in the form of their pampering, spoilt-for-choice and assistance with preparations for her coming baby, made it all a memorable experience. She admits that the same cannot be said about her second pregnancy, by which time she was living in a nuclear set-up in a different city.

With young people moving to new cities, often for employment opportunities, they start planning their future in small, nuclear families, to suit their lifestyle. The efforts to maintain a balance between career and personal goals have been in the discussion from the beginning of this decade. The importance of maintaining fitness via various activities—be it the gym, dance classes, aerobics or yoga—has become paramount for maintaining this balance. With the stress factors including the rising cost of good education and health, the focus on earning enough and more has now increased multifold. Both partners prepare well and choose to bring in a baby and the ensuing new set of responsibilities as 'the ready couple'. This couple consciously takes the decision to step into parenthood and prepares for the onset of this new phase of life. They are more likely to have the finances, their personal time and career aspirations planned around the same for the coming years. Their health takes on more importance than usual and this is where yoga comes in.

Yoga exercises have often been advised to reduce the stress level in our lives. It is not surprising then that our age-old bank of knowledge has a few tips for this essential stage in a human's life—procreation. From preparing the body and mind to aiding it through the drastic changes, to the healing afterwards, yoga has proved to be a safe and healthy exercise in this restless world. It works on the stress which comes with the changes one experiences while preparing and healing the body through any and all problems that may occur.

The following pages will take you through the various exercises for each stage of the change, from preparing your body and mind before you embark on this journey of conception to the post-pregnancy care and the road back to recovery through fitness. It is strongly recommended that all exercises be performed only if your doctor deems you fit for them. Putting any undue strain on your body is not advised.

1

Get Started

It's a good idea to visit your doctor when you start planning for a family. Health check-ups have become a norm these days but when one wants to increase the chances of conception, a visit to your doctor is strongly advised. Booking a pre-pregnancy check-up at your gynaecologist at least three months before you plan to start trying, will help you stay up-to-date on vaccinations, checked for STDs (sexually transmitted diseases), making sure that any chronic conditions such as diabetes, asthma, or thyroid problems are in check, and you are tested for heart-health issues like high blood pressure and cholesterol. Keeping a check on your body functions and the knowledge that everything is normal improves your chances of conception. Several young couples in their thirties consult me about their health, where the woman is suffering from PCOS (Polycystic Ovary Syndrome) or the male has a low sperm count, being underweight or overweight, with unhealthy lifestyles. These are hindrances and need to be addressed if the couple wants to start a family.

Contraceptives

Misuse of contraceptives is a rampant problem. And the only solution, I believe, is more awareness of their drawbacks. Their side effects show up in later stages of life. Instances are abound of early unplanned pregnancies that cannot be carried through. It is thus very important to meet up with your family doctor or your GP (general physician) on a regular basis to understand the best contraceptive measures.

Women who have been on the contraceptive pill for years don't realize what they have put their body through. The first sign of overdoing contraceptive pills for years at a stretch is irregular periods. Women should take the time to read and weigh the cons while choosing medication or products. Just going by the advertisements for such pills is not advised as the advertisements are meant for awareness of such products but their intake should be prescribed by your doctor.

Common Contraceptive Measures

1. **Oestrogen and Progesterone Pills (EnPs):** Doctor-prescribed POPs are to be taken at the same time every day. It interferes with ovulation and/or sperm function.
2. **Condoms:** Available both for men and woman. Most popular form of contraception as it protects against STDs as well.
3. **Emergency Contraception Pill:** Hormonal pills which are taken either as a single dose or two doses 12 hours apart in the event of unprotected sex. It should not be used as a regular contraceptive method.

Easier access to information through the Internet often opens up unwanted doors for young people, who may be unaware of the consequences of certain decisions. I still remember a time when we had a strict time schedule for playing and watching TV. There were certain programmes and movies that had the minimum age specified, and we knew it wasn't meant for us. But parental control is almost obsolete now. The kids' concept of fun and entertainment has ceased to remain innocent. They look up to role-models like actors and virtual characters and emulate their dressing, lifestyle and so on. All this can have an adverse effect on them. Experimenting with over-the-counter medication which is often advertised on TV and exposure to explicit content on the free Internet has often led to unintended harmful activities by youngsters.

Let me give you an example: 14-year-old Glory was from an orthodox family, who did a lot of social work. Glory was raised with good values and lived a happy-go-lucky life. She always ranked first in academics as well as sports. As Glory entered her teenage days, she became very self-conscious about her body and appearance. A natural process when youth blossoms; puberty brought in breasts, pubic hair and periods. She was attracted to the opposite sex, something she couldn't discuss with her parents and siblings. Glory studied in a convent school that frowned upon even interacting with boys. But breaking rules and exploring is part of being a teenager.

Glory befriended James, who was from the same community. An attractive boy, James was the quintessential cool kid, good at sports. Everyone wanted to be his friend and hang out with him. Glory would notice him often and smile and walk past him. After some time, James proposed to Glory, asking her to be his girlfriend. Glory was thrilled but shy and told him she would need time to make a decision. All of Glory's friends told her she would be considered crazy if she refused his proposal, as he was the most popular boy. Finally, she conceded and they got into a relationship. Unlike the times of her grandparents, where even holding a girl's hand—leave alone a peck on the cheek—would take months to come around, everything seemed to be on the fast track. James wanted to take the relationship further and insisted to Glory that their proclaimed love meant they could take their relationship to the next level. Glory, fearing she would lose James, finally gave in.

James would use a condom every now and then, but a boy his age couldn't blow up all his pocket money on those. He tried to convince her that it was okay to have sex without a condom, or any other method of contraception. Glory was still scared as she remembered the sex education class she had been to and decided to take things into her own hands. Thereafter, to have safe sex, Glory resorted to emergency contraceptive pills, aka the morning-after pill. She searched for an ad she had noticed on TV about a pill. Instead of going to a gynaecologist and educating herself, Glory chose the most convenient alternative to safe sex. As Glory didn't know the inherent risks of misusing emergency contraceptive pills, it became her regular safety resort.

The number of people using emergency contraceptive pills is rising at a rapid rate and the sad thing is that the buyers are not aware of the side effects or long-term effects of these pills.

Some of the most common scenarios doctors come across in such cases of rampant pill usage are irregular periods or failed attempts to prevent pregnancy. In this case, Glory was lucky that her relationship ended before things got worse, but little did Glory know how she had adversely compromised her body and health. The morning-after pill is not to be misused. It should only be taken in an emergency, such as when a condom breaks. There are too many cases of youth misusing these pills which are so easily available. I know of cases where these pills are taken as many as five times in the same month. This is dangerous for the health of the woman. Also, it is important to keep in mind, if not taken in time, that is, within the 72-hour stipulation, the failure rate gets higher as time passes.

I strongly recommend using a condom every time. It will protect you from any STI (sexually transmitted infection) and STDs such as chlamydia and gonorrhoea, a major cause of infertility, all high-risk today, as it is not uncommon for people to have had multiple partners. Once an individual contracts an STI, it can be life-threatening. If you wish to conceive later, STIs could affect the baby as well. So, it is very important to choose the best method for you.

PURPOSE OF A BIRTH CONTROL PILL

To help us better understand, judge and opt for them, it is important to know the constitution of birth control pills. The popular ones are a combination of two hormones—oestrogen and progesterone—that have been altered minutely in molecular structure from the body's natural hormones and convey vastly different biological messages and effects. Basically, they trick the reproductive system. They prevent the release of eggs from ovaries. It also thickens the mucus in the cervical area that blocks the passage of sperms.

This happened with Muskan—a girl happily married to her high-school sweetheart, Sanjay. Before getting married, they were committed and shared a healthy and an open-dialogue relationship with their parents, who accepted their relationship as long as it didn't affect their academics, and they observed certain boundaries and rules. Muskan got on the pill. She kept a reminder on her mobile phone that would ring every afternoon at 3 p.m. to remind her, as this contraceptive was advised to be taken at a certain time daily. Muskan and Sanjay had decided to get married once their careers took off and Sanjay was financially independent.

A few years later, Sanjay, now 30 years old and Muskan, 29, got married. Their plan was to settle down, buy a house and then have children. Sanjay knew at that time he would soon accomplish these goals, and within two years, they were able to buy a house. Sanjay and Muskan were happy and they agreed that it was time Muskan left her job. She had always wanted to be a stay-at-home wife, and focus all her attention on her husband and kids. She was still on the pill. Ready to plan a baby, she decided to get off it. She spot-bled soon after, and her periods were irregular. They tried to conceive naturally but were unsuccessful for a year. Muskan felt depressed and doubted if she was even fit to become a mother. When she contacted her gynaecologist, he explained that some women get pregnant soon after whereas some women's bodies take time to adjust to the sudden change. Since she began using birth control very young, the chances of getting pregnant within the first year of discontinuing the contraceptive pill depended on her health.

Muskan took things into her own hands. Back in the day, the elders would arrange for a doctor when they recognized the signs and symptoms of pregnancy, and on confirmation, some of the elders who were much experienced in this field played the role of mid-wives. A woman would specifically visit a doctor only when the symptoms did not convince the elders and her. Whatever form of birth control you adopt, a thorough check-up is advised before planning a pregnancy, to get necessary blood tests, update immunizations, vitamin supplements, and lifestyle changes like quitting smoking and alcohol, and losing weight, if necessary.

There are cases where women get pregnant soon after they stop the pill. Some others may take a significantly longer time to get their body back to its normal ovulation cycle. The body usually restores its fertility state within a year or so. Underlying factors such as age, weight, or other physiological issues could be considered in cases where women do not start their regular period cycle after stopping the pill.

EFFECTS OF BEING ON THE PILL FOR TOO LONG

There are several side effects a woman can experience while on the pill. The pill interferes with natural body functions, impeding the cyclic, self-regulated rhythm. The chemistry of these external hormones is foreign to the body. And it is a given that some changes occur, damaging the body clock and altering optimum functionality, reversibly or irreversibly, depending on how well the individual's coping mechanism is. The chances of contracting sexually transmitted diseases in such a state are extremely high.

Youngsters or even adults these days, tend to have multiple sexual partners at some point in life, and these people stand a chance of contracting different infections, especially those who don't use condoms and prefer the pill. The pills don't safeguard you from this.

Many girls come to me with the history of an irregular menstrual cycle. One of the main reasons is missing or being on the pill for too long, disrupting their entire natural cycle. There are cases of girls who suffer from serious medical conditions like early ovarian failures, making them infertile and prone to early menopause. It is always best for young boys and girls to talk to elders or school counsellors, if not family members, about sex and educate themselves rather than resorting to random Internet information, word of mouth advice and tips.

Fertility

A menstrual cycle is something that most women need to really keep a track of once they reach adolescence. Women should keep a track of their periods for many health reasons, which usually give you signs if anything is wrong. For those who do not get their periods regularly, experience heavy bleeding (also known as menorrhagia), minimal bleeding, clots, not getting a period or missing by a few months (also known as secondary menorrhagia), painful periods and so on, should know that these are underlining problems and signs that need to be checked by a doctor. If you notice any change, immediately inform your doctor. The body sends signs through different ways like the symptoms above to make you aware that there is an underlying problem.

The menstrual cycle of a woman determines her reproductive health status. An average regular period cycle lasts for 28 days but I'm not saying that there is a problem if you experience a longer or shorter cycle, as many women even have 21 to 35-day cycles.

For many women, it is very confusing to keep a tab on their ovulation and fertile dates. It has become much easier today as kits to detect your ovulation are easily available in a chemist shop or you can even use mobile apps. You can identify your fertile window as the days of ovulation are usually 12 to 16 days before your menstrual cycle begins and the 5 days that follow. That would be any day from day 10 to day 17. Many women experience different durations in cycles, therefore, it is important for you to identify yours. There are different, natural ways also, to identify your fertility like using a basal thermometer and keeping a track of the days your temperature increases. Another way is keeping a track on your bodily fluid called mucus (after your period). It differs from being dry to sticky to wet to stringy/stretchy (almost transparent) during ovulation. You would usually ovulate two days prior to and two days after you feel the stretchy/ stringy mucus.

During ovulation, an ovum is released where an unfertilized egg can live for 12 to 24 hours before it dies, therefore, the window for pregnancy is very small for getting the timing right but that should not stress you out because a sperm can live up to 24- 36 hours depending on its health, which is enough to get a woman pregnant.

There are many factors for not getting pregnant even after calculation which could be due to mainly stress, illness, poor diet, lack of exercise or too much exertion. It is always best to visit your doctor and get a proper examination done to determine any problem before taking to the Internet and jumping to conclusions.

Infertility

Women in their 20s and 30s who have regular menstrual cycles might suddenly have delays as they age. It is very important to mention this to your doctor. With age, fertility decreases in both partners. Weight is a huge factor as well. To ensure your weight is in the optimum range for fertility, your BMI (Body Mass Index) should be between 18.5 and 24. Exercising for 30 to 60 minutes each day initially will help you jump-start and manage your weight.

Couples who wait long to conceive are likely to struggle to have kids as age is a huge factor of fertility. But even young couples today report infertility issues. This problem of infertility can be faced by either partner or both. We encounter cases where a lifestyle of moderation or abstinence with regard to drinking, smoking or drugs, still does not guarantee optimum fertility and then others where people exploit their body system and clock with other agents but are still able to get pregnant. So don't beat yourself over it! This only implies there are several factors that work in tandem to create the individual's reproductive health.

Most of us go through this waiting period and I was no exception. I got married in May 2009, and after a few months, my husband and I decided to have a baby as we both were 34. But it wasn't an easy road. We started trying in 2010, naturally, as advised by our doctor. We got all our tests done and everything was fine. I started with taking Folvite tablets as suggested by my gynaecologist, Dr Hemant Brahme, and he suggested that I try for 6 months naturally, which I did, but all in vain. Slowly, desperation and stress started taking a toll on me. Every month I would pray to get pregnant and hope every time that this was it and hope that I wouldn't get my periods, but I would and after 6 months of trying, every month was a torture. Every time I would see the negative sign on the test, it would make me very anxious and depressed. While all this was going on, I was in the process of writing my first book *From XL to XS*. After giving it some more time I started focusing all my energies on my book. My in-laws were staying with us during that time on their annual vacation. One day, I had just taken a test and left it in my bathroom when it showed up negative again. I still remember my hubby, Manish, walking into the bathroom, then walking out into the living room where all of us were sitting. He made eye-contact with me, signalling me to come to our bedroom. I clearly remember him sitting me down while he stood near the windows and explained to me, on a very spiritual level, that everything happens for a reason. He reminded me that I had written a letter to God with a list of things I want to do. Just like the book and other things happened and were slowly being ticked off, I had to give it time. My checklist was being ticked off one at a time, and at the right given time, a baby would come. Manish left for Latvia with Kareena Kapoor and Saif Ali Khan, and I visited the doctor. He detected that one of my tubes was blocked and even after doing a D&C (dilation and curettage) procedure, the chances were still low as only one tube was functional. I was quite taken aback and sad. He gave me a time span between which I should try and also think about other procedures like IVF (in vitro fertilization). This happened in September. I, then, had to fly off to Las Vegas for 20 days with Kareena. My doctor was upset with me as this was the best time for me to try. I had to choose work but I took my mother along with me as she is a theta healer and did a lot of internal healing on me. We were back in December and for New Year's, we took off to my brother-in-law's place in Hyderabad. After our return, I headed out on 15 January 2011, to Kaivalyadhama Institute in Lonavala, to do a further course in yoga. I had been planning to do that for a long time and finally had the opportunity. As we say, man proposes and God disposes but only for our good! Within ten days of the course, I realized I was finally pregnant!

Thus, I can confidently say that I know how stressful it can be during this time, but suggest that you sit and talk to your partner and visit a doctor together. Follow up on the check-up and test results, and the doctor's advice. Communicate with each other and work towards an integrated solution. There is no point stressing oneself out. The more you stress, the more difficult the process is going to be. During this time, both partners need to support each other. If one partner cannot handle the stress, I recommend you confide in someone close to you—a friend or parent or sibling. Open up because internalizing all these fears and emotions takes a toll on the human body, emotionally and physically. Do not isolate yourself or let your doubts get the best of you.

Infertility issues can take a huge toll on a relationship. Either of the partners could clamp up, but at such a time, it helps to discuss it. A good support system is essential. My generic observation is that because men are conditioned to put up a strong front and be less expressive, it may take a while to break through. It doesn't mean they are impervious to the same insecurities, even if they don't say it. It has been observed that fathers may feel displaced during the pre-pregnancy as well as early days of pregnancy because the mothers become the focus. The feelings of isolation in the father-to-be need to be addressed by initiating conversations and answering possible questions. It is thus essential to visit a GP to manage the emotional stress of couples trying to have a baby.

Don't turn to Google for answers; it is always best to visit your doctor and open up about everything as only then can the doctor fully understand the issue, and work towards helping you. Many couples, on learning about their low fertility levels, often jump to considering IVF as the only opportunity, not realizing that there are other ways. The IVF procedure costs a lot. All hope is not lost for those who cannot afford it, there are other tested methods one can try to have a child, like turning to yoga.

Common Problems Couples Face

One should stay in touch with a gynaecologist if problems relating to fertility persist. It can be a result of various issues, which are discussed below.

PERIOD PROBLEMS

This is a common problem. Pubescent girls are reported to have irregular period cycles with gaps extending for 3 to 6 months. But some women suffer from this when they're older due to other underlying issues. It could be that the endocrine glands aren't producing the stimulating hormones that release progesterone and oestrogen to the ovaries, through the pituitary glands. When the function of this entire cycle is disrupted for any reason, the imbalance causes problems in the menstrual cycle. There are a few yoga exercises one can do to on a regular basis to help when the period problems set in. These are strictly not to be performed during your period.

Warm up:
1. **Upper body twist, 10 counts:** Stand with legs slightly apart. Clasp the fingers behind the head. Press the elbows slightly back. During the whole exercise, the soles of the feet remain flat on the floor, and the upper body and head remain in a straight line. The legs remain straight during the twist. Inhale deeply. Exhaling, turn the upper body to the left. Inhaling, return to the centre. Exhaling, turn the upper body to the right. Inhaling, return to the centre.

2. **Arms stretching, 10 counts:** Extend one hand down the centre of your back, fingers pointing downwards. Use the other hand to grasp the fingers. Exhale slowly, pulling gently downwards on your elbow, aiming to take your fingers along your spine.

3. **Shoulder rotation, 10 counts:** Cross one arm horizontally over your chest, grasping it with either your hand or forearm, just above the elbow joint. Exhale, slowly pulling your upper arm towards your chest. Aim to keep the hips and shoulders facing forwards throughout the stretch.

4. **Neck stretch, 10 counts:** Incline your head forward, but do not roll your head from side to side—this is dangerous. Instead, stretch your neck to the left, right, upwards and downwards, but always return to the centre first! Tilt your head with an ear towards the shoulder, incline your head backwards and roll your head from left to right, then right to left in a 30-degree motion. Be sure that while your head is tilted back, you keep your jaw relaxed and even let your mouth fall open just a bit.

5. **Forward stretch, 10 counts:** Stand with your feet shoulder-width apart, one foot extended half a step forward. Keeping the front leg straight, bend your rear leg, resting both hands on the bent thigh. Slowly exhale, aiming to tilt both buttocks upwards, keeping the front leg straight, and both feet flat on the floor, pointing forward. Inhale slowly, and relax from this stretching exercise. Repeat the stretch again, this time beginning with the toes of the front foot raised towards the ceiling, but keeping the heel on the floor.

6. **Backward stretch, 10 counts:** Stand with feet hip-width apart and toes pointed forward. Reach both arms out in

front of you and clasp your hands together. Now reach your arms out in front of you and turn your palms to face forwards. Hold this stretch for about 30 seconds.

7. **Upward stretch, 10 counts:** Extend both hands straight above your head, palms touching. Inhale, slowly pushing your hands upwards, then downwards, keeping your back straight. Exhale while relaxing from the stretch before you repeat.

8. **Side stretch, 10 counts:** Stand with your feet together and your arms straight overhead. Clasp your hands together, with your fingers interlocked and pointer fingers extended. Inhale as you reach upwards. Breathe out as you bend your upper body to the right. Take 5 slow breaths. Slowly return to the centre. Repeat on the left side.

9. **Leg stretch, 10 counts:** Stand holding onto a secure object, or have one hand raised out to the side for balance. Raise one heel up towards your buttocks, and grasp your foot with one hand. Inhale, slowly pulling your heel to your buttock while gradually pushing your pelvis forward. Aim to keep both knees together, having a slight bend in the supporting leg.

10. **Wrist rotation, 10 counts:** Sit on the floor, legs stretched out straight before you, hands resting on your thighs. Close your eyes and breathe deeply for a few moments to prepare for the wrist rotation yoga exercises. Stretch your arms out straight in front of you, though be careful not to hyperextend at the elbows. With your arms stretched out straight, close your hands into fists, with your thumbs tucked inside. You need not clench. The fists should be loose and comfortable. Slowly rotate your fists at the wrists—

your right fist completing circles in a clockwise motion and your left fist completing circles in a counter-clockwise motion. Complete 10 rotations. Switch the direction of each fist's rotation—your right fist now moving in a counter-clockwise motion and your left fist now moving in a clockwise motion. Complete 10 rotations.

The asanas are as follows and should be performed on 10–15 counts three times:

Tadasana

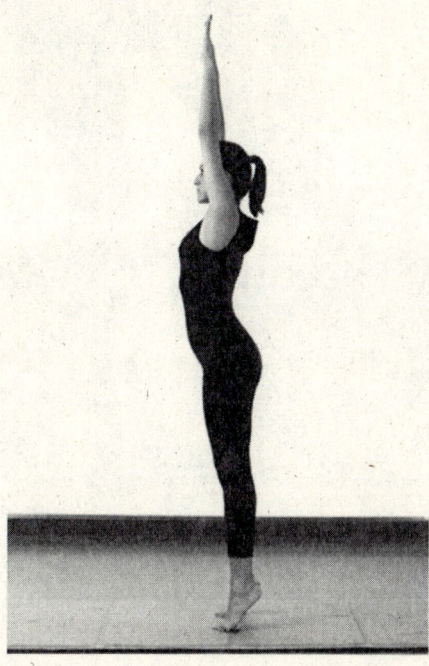

Stand straight with your feet shoulder-width apart, and your hands to the side of your body. Inhale slowly, raising your hands upwards with your palms facing out. Stretch your entire body while standing on your toes. In the final position hold for some time, breathing normally. Come down to the original position slowly, while exhaling.

Benefits: Improves height and flexibility of the spine and stretches the calves and tones the buttocks.

Padahastasana

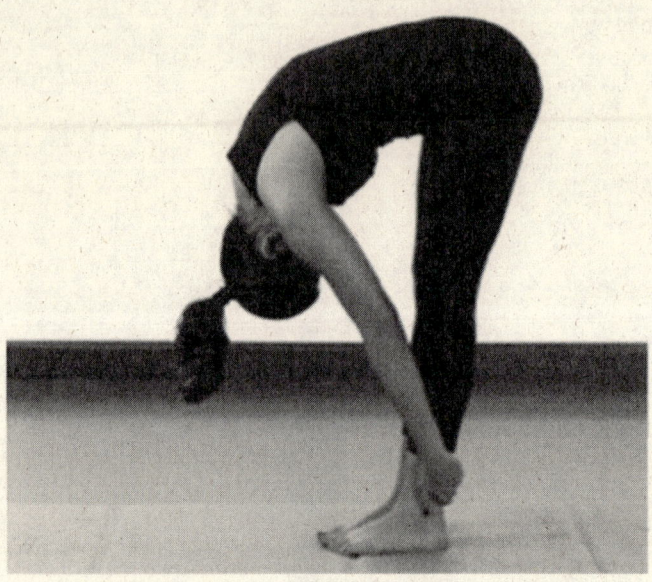

Stand straight with your feet together and hands by the side of your body. While inhaling, raise your hands up and then, while exhaling, bend the body forward from the hip and try to touch your toes with your fingers without bending your knees. Look downwards and breathe normally once you are in this posture.

Benefits: Improves flexibility of the hamstrings and lower back.

Janushirshasana

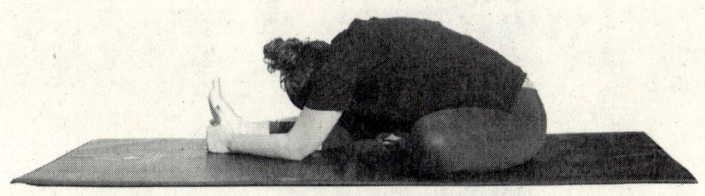

Sit on the floor with both legs stretched out in front of you. Keep the back straight and the hands by the side. Bend your right knee and place your right foot on the inner thigh of the left leg. Inhale and raise both hands upwards, and then exhale slowly, bending forward, and hold the ankle of the left leg. Try and place your forehead on the left knee and try and touch the elbows to the floor. Hold it there for some time, breathing normally. Repeat the same with the other leg.

Benefits: Reduces fat from the abdomen and increases the flexibility of the back.

Ushtrasana

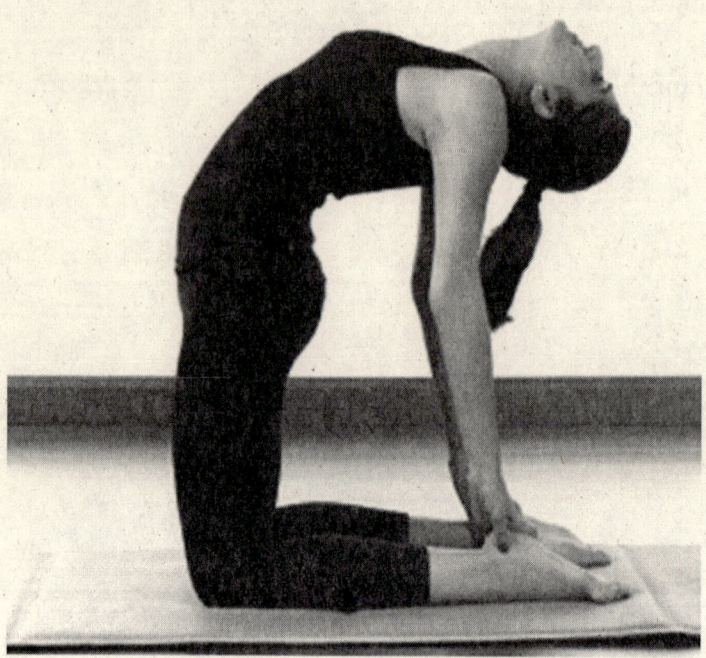

Sit straight in Vajrasana. Slowly stand on the knees, keeping them shoulder-width apart. Now slowly turn your upper body to the right and try to touch the right heel with the right hand, and the left heel with the left hand while balancing the body. After holding the heels, inhale and push the waist forward and drop the neck back. Breathe normally in the final position. Hold for some time. While exhaling, come back to the normal position.

Benefits: Removes stiffness from the thighs, abdomen, chest, shoulders, arms and neck muscles.

Paschimottanasana

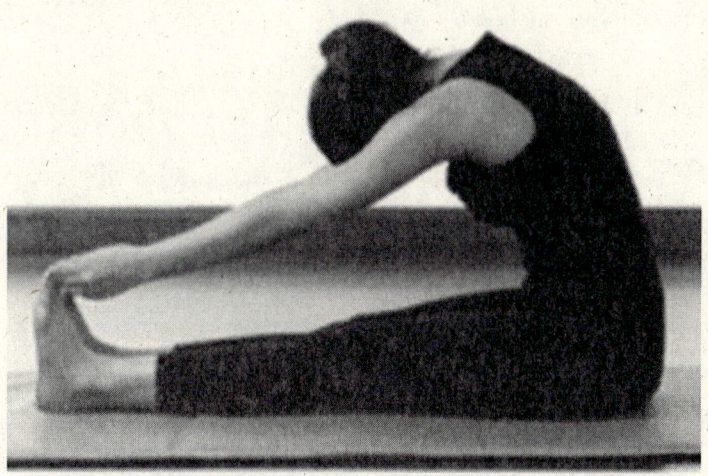

Sit on the floor with your legs stretched out straight and your palms on your thighs, keeping your heels on the floor. Inhale and take your hands upwards with your palms facing each other. Now bend forward and try to hold your big toe with your two fingers without bending your knees towards you. Keep bending forward as much as you can, while trying to touch your knees with your nose. Hold this for some time, breathing normally, and then slowly come back to the original position. Initially, one may not be flexible enough to get into this posture as the fat in the abdomen may act as a barrier. Nonetheless, at the initial stage bend as much as you can, but don't bend your knees. Don't do it too fast, as it is more important to remain in the bending posture for a longer duration, than doing it for an increased number of times.

Benefits: Tones and massages the abdomen and pelvic region, stretches the back and hamstring muscles and increases flexibility in the hip.

Pawanmukthasana

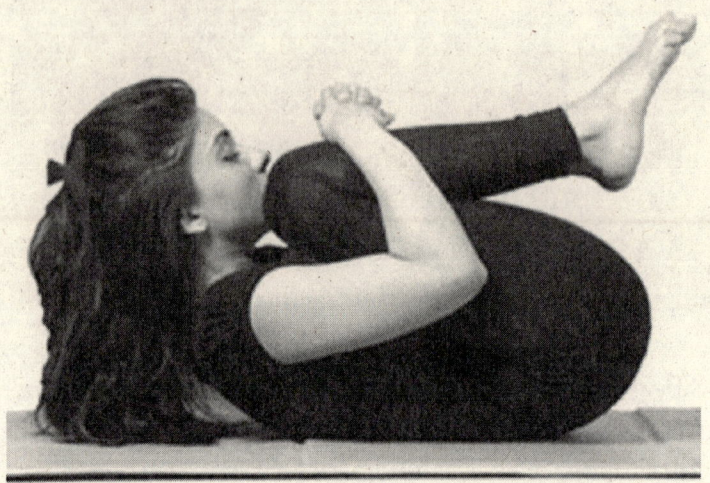

Lie in a supine position with your legs together, hands by the side, and palms resting on the floor. Slowly bend both knees together towards the chest. Hold your knees with your hands and pull towards the chest. Raise your chin up between the knees, and hold for some time, breathing normally. Then come back to the original position.

Benefits: Helps with acidity, constipation, headache and low blood pressure.

Marjariasana

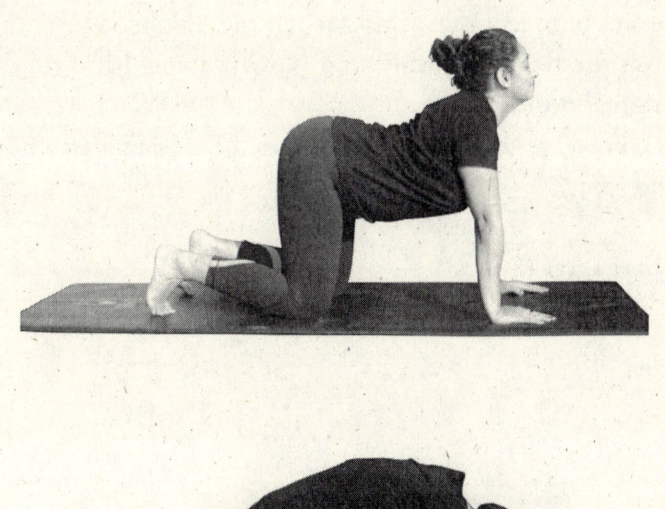

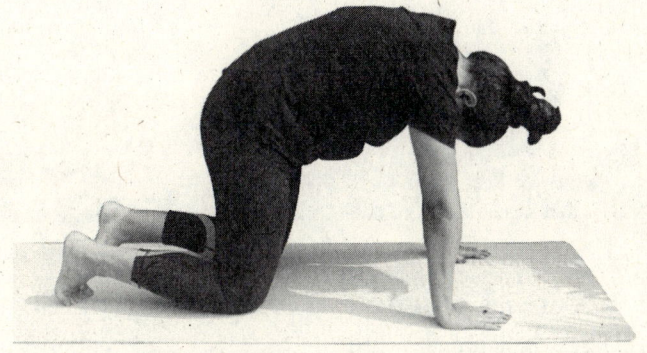

Come in a cat position on the mat. Now inhale while raising the head upwards and pushing the back downwards, and make a major contraction on the buttock muscles. Hold for some time. Exhale while lowering the head and stretching the spine upwards. The head will now be in between the arms facing the thighs. Hold this position for some time and slowly come back to the original position.

Benefits: Improves flexibility in the shoulders, neck and spine.

Sharnagrat Mudra

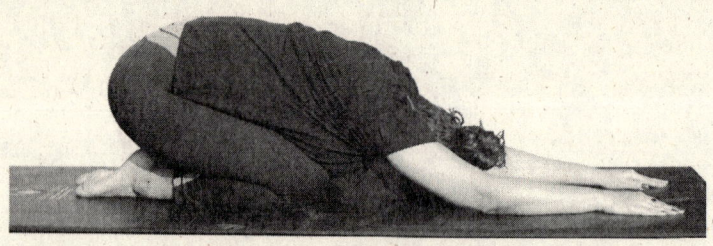

Sit in Vajrasana with the back straight. Slowly inhale and raise both the hands upwards. Now exhale, and bend forward slowly. Touch your palms on the floor by stretching the arms but without bending the elbows. Now place your head on the floor with the abdomen pressed to the thighs. Do not raise the buttocks. Hold this position.

Benefits: Improves digestive functions.

Shavasana

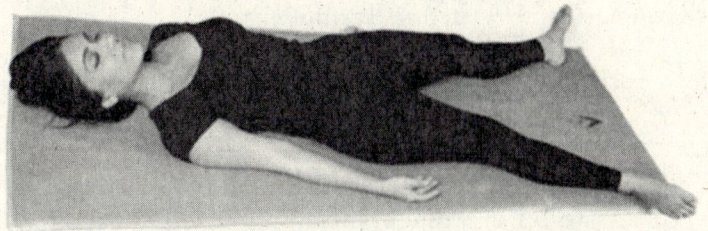

Lie down on the back with the legs together and hands on the side. Spread the legs apart slowly, with your heels facing one another and toes pointing outside. Keep your hands away from the body, with the palms facing upwards. Close your eyes and relax all the muscles in your body and focus on breathing.

Benefits: Removes fatigue from the body and relaxes all muscles.

RECOVERY FROM BIRTH CONTROL ISSUES

Birth control medications and artificial hormones disrupt the menstrual cycle. They play a huge role in causing a shift in the natural process of bodily functions, adversely affecting the uterus, thinning its lining. It usually takes a whole year for your body to restore normalcy, flush out these physiological changes and regulate smooth functioning. Many women take hormone-induced medication for related concerns like PCOS (Polycystic

Ovarian Syndrome), fertility and other menstrual issues. It is important not to confuse them with birth control hormones, as they are totally different.

PCOS

When the hormonal balance of the body is affected, it leads to many issues in women, including PCOS. I encounter many such cases where women try to reverse side effects which range from affecting fertility to unwanted facial and body hair growth, acne, thinning of hair on the head, weight gain, trouble in losing weight, unexplainable depression and skin outbreaks. If not treated, this could cause a huge long-term problem that could trigger other health issues.

THYROID

There are two kinds of effects: Hyper and Hypo. It is basically the overproduction or underproduction of the thyroid hormone resulting in an imbalance. An overactive thyroid gland causes Hyperthyroidism and an underactive thyroid gland results in Hypothyroidism.

People with Hyperthyroidism experience weight loss, excessive sweating, palpitations, rapid heart rate, problems in concentrating, fatigue, change in hair texture making it thinner and brittle, and irregular menstrual flow. Hypothyroidism causes unexplained weight gain, dry skin, increased sensitivity to cold, hair loss, goitre, a change in bowel movements, among other problems.

If not treated properly or ignored, both conditions could cause infertility, heart-related problems, obesity-related complications, to name a few.

Preparing for Pregnancy Physically and Mentally

TACKLING DIFFERENT WEIGHT ISSUES
(Underweight/ideal weight/overweight/obese)

Women who plan to conceive are always advised about their weight. Those who are overweight or obese need to work on themselves before getting pregnant, as it sometimes could affect both the baby and the mother.

Those who suffer from obesity or are overweight also have lower production of the prolactin hormone, which helps in lactation. Many overweight women these days stop producing milk earlier than a healthy ideal weight woman. To avoid such problems, a woman should be at, or close to, her ideal weight, if possible, when she becomes pregnant. My advice for women is to lose at least 5–10 per cent of their body weight before getting pregnant so it is easier on the mother as well as the baby, negating many risks inherent in overweight pregnancies. But since not every pregnancy is planned, any overweight woman who becomes pregnant is usually motivated to improve her health and weight to avoid any complications. That being said, there is no cause for undue concern. You could safely continue your pregnancy with a few adjustments here and there. Doctors advise all women to put on or gain anything between 8 and 15 kg during pregnancy.

In the case of overweight or obese women, they usually already have a greater store of the nutrients a developing baby needs.

HOW TO CALCULATE IF ONE IS OVERWEIGHT OR UNDERWEIGHT?

A Body Mass Index (BMI, a formula that relates weight to height) of 25 to 29.9 is considered overweight, while a BMI greater than 30 is the current standard for obesity. Dr Hemant Brahme says, 'BMI is a good indicator of the overall health of an individual. BMI within normal range means stable hormonal status, less oxidative stress and more organ productivity, including gonads. Needless to say, the fertility of an individual and the BMI have a cause-and-effect relationship!'

WEIGHT IN KILOGRAMS

Height in Centimetres

	45	48	50	53	55	58	60	63	65	68	70	73	75	78	80	82.5	85	87.5	90
145.0	21.4	22.6	23.8	25.0	26.2	27.3	28.5	29.7	30.9	32.1	33.3	34.5	35.7	36.9	38.0	39.2	40.4	41.6	42.8
147.5	20.7	21.8	23.0	24.1	25.3	26.4	27.6	28.7	29.9	31.0	32.2	33.3	34.5	35.6	36.8	37.9	39.1	40.2	41.4
150.0	20.0	21.1	22.2	23.3	24.4	25.6	26.7	27.8	28.9	30.0	31.1	32.2	33.3	34.4	35.6	36.7	37.8	38.9	40.0
152.5	19.3	20.4	21.5	22.6	23.6	24.7	25.8	26.9	27.9	29.0	30.1	31.2	32.2	33.3	34.4	35.5	36.5	37.6	38.7
155.0	18.7	19.8	20.8	21.9	22.9	23.9	25.0	26.0	27.1	28.1	29.1	30.2	31.2	32.3	33.3	34.3	35.4	36.4	37.5
157.5	18.1	19.1	20.2	21.2	22.2	23.2	24.2	25.2	26.2	27.2	28.2	29.2	30.2	31.2	32.2	33.3	34.3	35.3	36.3
160.0	17.6	18.6	19.5	20.5	21.5	22.5	23.4	24.4	25.4	26.4	27.3	28.3	29.3	30.3	31.3	32.2	33.2	34.2	35.2
162.5	17.0	18.0	18.9	19.9	20.8	21.8	22.7	23.7	24.6	25.6	26.5	27.5	28.4	29.3	30.3	31.2	32.2	33.1	34.1
166.0	16.5	17.4	18.4	19.3	20.2	21.1	22.0	23.0	23.9	24.8	25.7	26.6	27.5	28.5	29.4	30.3	31.2	32.1	33.1
167.5	16.0	16.9	17.8	18.7	19.6	20.5	21.4	22.3	23.2	24.1	24.9	25.8	26.7	27.6	28.5	29.4	30.3	31.2	32.1
170.0	15.6	16.4	17.3	18.2	19.0	19.9	20.8	21.6	22.5	23.4	24.2	25.1	26.0	26.8	27.7	28.5	29.4	30.3	31.1
172.5	15.1	16.0	16.8	17.6	18.5	19.3	20.2	21.0	21.8	22.7	23.5	24.4	25.2	26.0	26.9	27.7	28.6	29.4	30.2
175.0	14.7	15.5	16.3	17.1	18.0	18.8	19.6	20.4	21.2	22.0	22.9	23.7	24.5	25.3	26.1	26.9	27.8	28.6	29.4
177.5	14.3	15.1	15.9	16.7	17.5	18.3	19.0	19.8	20.6	21.4	22.2	23.0	23.8	24.6	25.4	26.2	27.0	27.8	28.6
180.0	13.9	14.7	15.4	16.2	17.0	17.7	18.5	19.3	20.1	20.8	21.6	22.4	23.1	23.9	24.7	25.5	26.2	27.0	27.8
182.5	13.5	14.3	15.0	15.8	16.5	17.3	18.0	18.8	19.5	20.3	21.0	21.8	22.5	23.3	24.0	24.8	25.5	26.3	27.0
185.0	13.1	13.9	14.6	15.3	16.1	16.8	17.5	18.3	19.0	19.7	20.5	21.2	21.9	22.6	23.4	24.1	24.8	25.6	26.3
187.5	12.8	13.5	14.2	14.9	15.6	16.4	17.1	17.8	18.5	19.2	19.9	20.6	21.3	22.0	22.8	23.5	24.2	24.9	25.6
190.0	12.5	13.2	13.9	14.5	15.2	15.9	16.6	17.3	18.0	18.7	19.4	20.1	20.8	21.5	22.2	22.9	23.5	24.2	24.9

Underweight   Normal   Overweight   Obesity

Some of the complications which may arise if the would-be mother is over-weight are:

- Hypertension: high blood pressure
- Pre-eclampsia: is a combination of hypertension, proteinuria, oedema or excess water in tissues, and characterized by swelling of feet and hands.
- Gestational diabetes: which can lead to overly large babies.
- C-section deliveries
- Post-operative complications

Doctors advise against losing weight during pregnancy because it might affect the mother's health, along with risking the health of the baby. It is necessary to be cautious about not limiting the intake of carbohydrates for rapid weight loss during pregnancy or resorting to high protein diets, which could, in turn, affect your foetus. A balanced, calorie-restricted, high-nutrient diet, on the other hand, can result in weight loss without causing any harm to the body and foetus.

STRESS

Stress causes insomnia. As they plan a pregnancy, both partners need to relax and enjoy this time. Couples can go on a vacation as that really helps. One thing I would like to emphasize here is, *do not* stress if you don't succeed as it might seem like friends and other people around you are getting pregnant easily.

Kapil and Shruti, married for six years and both successful in their careers in the finance industry, decided to have a child. They visited their doctor and got their tests where everything proved to be normal. Excited about this, they started trying to conceive. Their regular lives continued along with the sometimes long hours and the irregular eating habits while on official tours. When, after more than seven months of trying they weren't able to conceive, they asked their doctor what could be wrong. After talking to them about their lifestyle, the doctor told them that they were simply too stressed out. The doctor advised them to take a vacation and consciously reduce the daily stress in their lives to improve their chances of conceiving. Eleven months later, they walked into the doctor's clinic with two positive pregnancy tests in hand.

CUT DOWN ON CAFFEINE INTAKE

Women shouldn't consume more than 200 mg of caffeine in a day. Too much of chocolate is also bad as 50 g of plain chocolate can contain as much as 50 mg of caffeine while one can of any soda contains 40 mg.

FOOD

Eating a healthy diet rich in vitamins and nutrients is the foundation of a healthy pregnancy. The diet of the mother during these months plays a huge role in the growth of the baby. Our entire hormonal system functions around the food we eat. There are many food items that have an effect on fertility and help boost it.

With my clients, the first thing I ask of them is to write down their daily schedules, listing the time they wake up till they hit the bed at night, to the food intake with the timings, and activities throughout the day. Thereafter, I sit and note the mistakes they make during the day and educate them as to how much it is affecting their lives. The next step is to make healthier changes gradually. Next, I get them to make their meals small and healthy. If both partners work and live independently, they find it difficult to cook daily. Their first interpretation of my suggested diet plan is a weight loss diet, but not all regimes have to be a crash or liquid diet. Start off with a healthy nutritious diet and then gradually move on to a body detox programme. This way the body doesn't go into shock and gradually adapts to the good change. Then I suggest fertility boosting diets which are based on specific nutrient-rich food items which are extremely good for women and men. They help with smooth functioning of body systems, clear all blockages, boost fertility and ensure optimum production and balance in the hormonal system.

The food in such diets contains more fibre, carbohydrates, proteins, fewer meats, and more fruit and vegetables, with multivitamins, and is rich in iron and calcium. It may also cut down drastically on sugar, caffeine and trans-fats (margarine, shortening and vegetable oil that's been hydrogenated).

Calcium is very important as it helps regulate heart rhythm while preventing blood clotting and muscle contraction. It also helps the formation of the baby's teeth and bones. It also lowers the risk of pre-eclampsia, a serious condition affecting pregnant women. The best sources are skimmed milk, low-fat yoghurt, calcium-fortified orange juice or soy milk, broccoli and so on.

Food containing Vitamin D boosts your immune system and mood. It is required for the baby's bone and teeth development. Many women don't consume the required amount of Vitamin D, especially those who don't drink milk. By staying indoors most of the day or even the use of sunscreen daily, deprives the mother of the natural calcium intake from the sun's rays.

The best source of Vitamin D is the sun. Bask for 10 to 15 minutes in the direct sun without any sunscreen or creams and with maximum body exposure during the time. Milk, eggs and cereals are rich in Vitamin D. Fish liver oil capsules (including cod and salmon) are excellent options. Many other supplements are also available.

For women to combat PCOS, regulating the diet as above and small lifestyle change ensures a huge improvement in health.

Yoga in Months before Pregnancy

During the months you plan to conceive, I suggest yoga routines with a focus on boosting fertility. Aside from the numerous benefits, the bonus is you can enjoy a better sex life. It relaxes the body and mind, keeping you calm and composed. It helps increase circulation to the main areas of the pelvis, working on internal organs, helping in raising the levels of hormones. Yoga helps build stamina and flexibility, sustaining you longer and making different positions more enjoyable.

Fertility yoga aims at increasing the energy flow through your body and thus improving the functions of the endocrine and reproductive systems. It uses a specific series of stretches that have a positive effect on reproductive health. The kind of exercise routine that I usually advise before pregnancy is not at all like the regular high-intensity workouts. Here we take things slow and work on the internal body. Yoga is the best option along with other forms of activities like jogging, swimming, brisk walking, Pilates. But in any workout, you need to keep a slow pace, remembering not to overwork the body. Remember you are preparing for pregnancy and not training for the Olympics.

Always get a good professional teacher to guide you instead of self-help, as at this time, it is very important how you get into or even hold your postures, be it in yoga or Pilates or a light gym workout, because by overdoing it or without proper guidance, you could hurt yourself, damaging your body and aggravating the condition further, making it difficult during pregnancy. Walking, yoga and swimming are excellent choices.

Benefits of Yoga

With regular yoga sessions and a healthy diet, there are innumerous health benefits one can receive. Here are a few that yoga can help with:

1. Hypothyroidism
2. Hormonal imbalances

3.   Absence of periods/irregular periods
4.   PCOS
5.   Recovery from birth control issues
6.   Infertility brought on by age and other underlying issues pertaining to infertility
7.   Men's fertility
8.   Miscarriages
9.   Ovarian cyst
10. Cervical mucus
11. Health of the eggs
12. Stress affecting fertility
13. Premature ovarian failure
14. Preparation for an IVF
15. Unexplained infertility
16. Low progesterone

PRENATAL YOGA

During this time the doctor might advise you to do yoga as it is the best form of preparing yourself for what is to come. Working on each pose and learning the conscious meaning of breathing the right way helps manage contractions during labour, making it easier for you and the baby.

Yoga is very important for the body balance during this time as the body isn't accustomed to weight gain. The constant overdrive by the body working on the development and growth of the baby puts a strain on you, making you tired, dizzy and wobbly. Yoga helps to bring about a balance. It helps increase stamina and endurance. That helps with your ability to carry the growing belly without getting tired too soon and helps perform normal chores with ease. Yoga helps in easing pain and swelling in the body. It helps in increasing circulation, keeping your blood pressure regulated.

There are many postures that help you stretch and relieve the stress and high amount of tension on your growing belly, hips and breasts. These put a tremendous strain on your back, neck, hips and legs. Work on good breathing techniques and supportive stretches, guided by a qualified yoga instructor.

In the meditation sessions for pregnant women at my studio, many mothers say that they experience a connection with their babies during such sessions. They are able to focus on the baby and their bodies at the same time, which is very important. As you inhale in a posture, you feel calm and composed, while exhaling de-stresses, causing a very positive effect on your baby, keeping you calm and connected. Personally, since I have been doing yoga for a long time, I have noticed that it eases out many discomforts during labour naturally. My body was more prepared for the hours of strenuous labour.

Another reason why I strongly recommend yoga for pregnancy is that women put a huge strain on their backs while carrying their growing bellies. That causes backaches that persist post-delivery when you need to carry your baby in your arms. Yoga helps stretch your back, giving it room to adapt to the changes gradually and making it easy to go about doing your motherly duties with ease. Yoga plays a huge role in the entire blood circulatory system, keeping swellings, aches and pains at bay, along with getting you back in shape after delivery. It works on firming up the muscles in your core, toning up the stomach once again, and also restoring the pelvis flow, which is usually weak after delivery.

One of the most effective asanas after pregnancy is Mula Bandha. It is somewhat similar to Kegel exercises—where you contract your vaginal muscles—but more effective. While passing urine, try the stop-and-go method. This helps during, as well as after, labour to control and hold your urine, as the elasticity in that area is also weak after delivery.

My sessions consist of workouts related to hormonal balance, fertility, regulating menstrual cycles, clearing blockages in the reproductive system, strengthening and improving circulation in the pelvis area. Some of the workouts are shared later in the chapter.

YOGA FOR BEGINNERS

1. **Warm-up Exercises** (see p. 14)

2. Suryanamaskar

a. Position: **Namaskar Mudra**

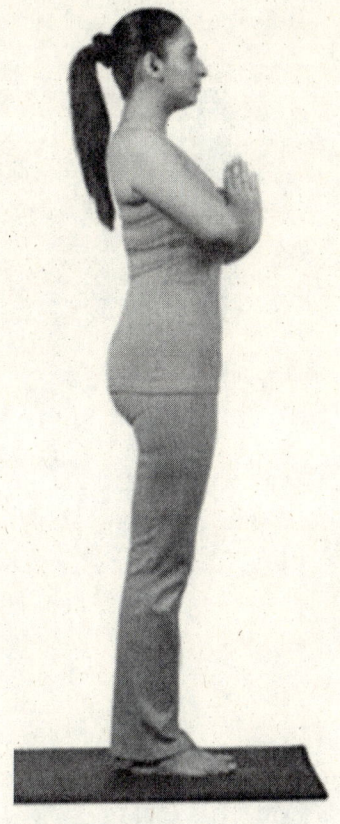

Stand straight with the feet together with hands by the side. Now put your palms together in Namaskar Mudra close to your chest. Breathe normally.

b.   Position: **Chakrasana**

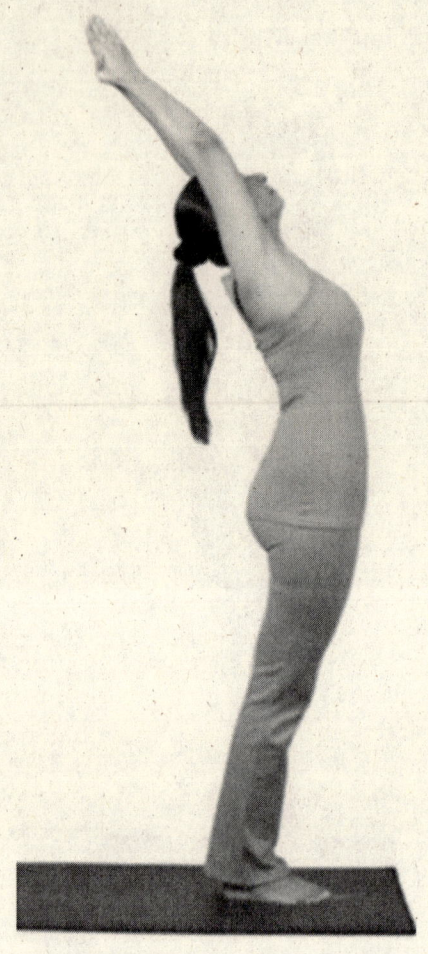

Inhale and raise your hands upwards; arch your back. Stretch your arms upwards as much as you can. Once in position, breathe normally.

c. Position: **Padahastasana**

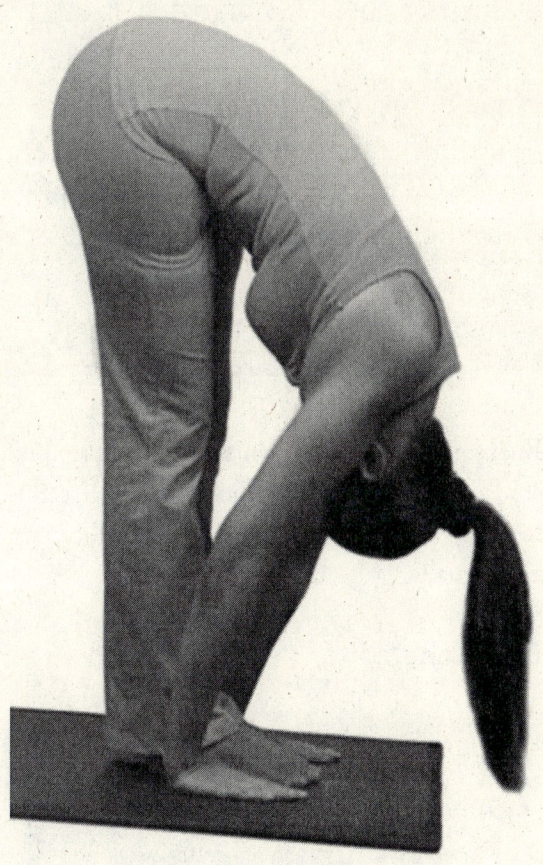

Now exhale and bend forward, touching your toes with your hands without bending your knees, drop your neck and breathe normally once in the posture.

d. Position: **Ashwa Sanchalanasana**

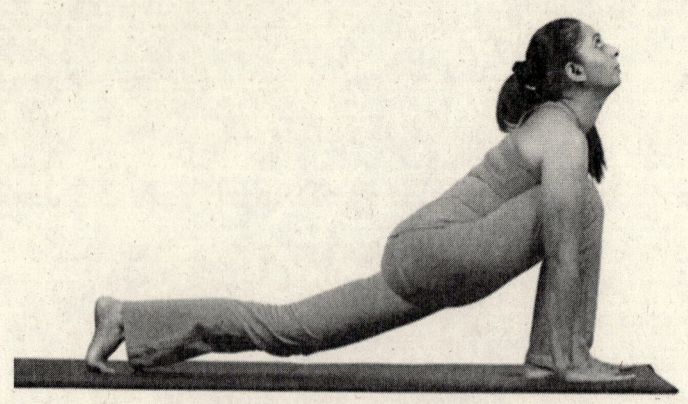

While inhaling put the palms on the floor, take the left leg behind and stretch back. Bend the right leg at a 90-degree angle from the floor, arch the back and look upwards, breathing normally.

e. Position: **Santolasana**

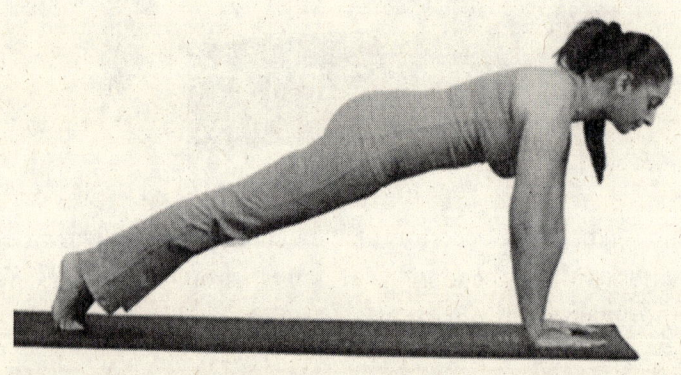

Exhale and put your right leg behind with the other leg. Make sure your hands are under the shoulders. The shoulders, back and hips should be in one line, parallel to the floor and once in the posture, breathe normally.

f.   Position: **Sashtanga Mudra**

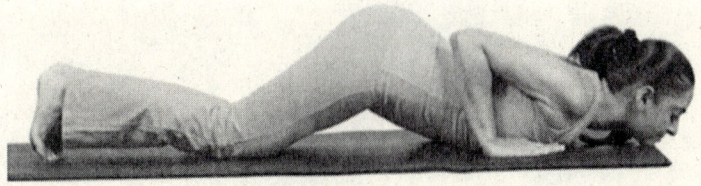

Bend your elbows, chin, chest and knees on the floor, tuck the elbows inside close to the body and raise your hips upwards, breathing normally.

g.   Position: **Sarpasana**

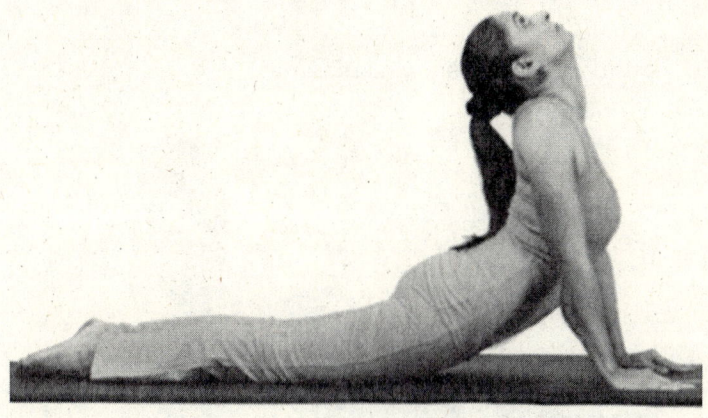

Inhale and raise your upper body, elbow straight, shoulders back, chin upwards and waist touching the floor. Once in the final posture, breathe normally.

h.   Position: **Parvatasana**

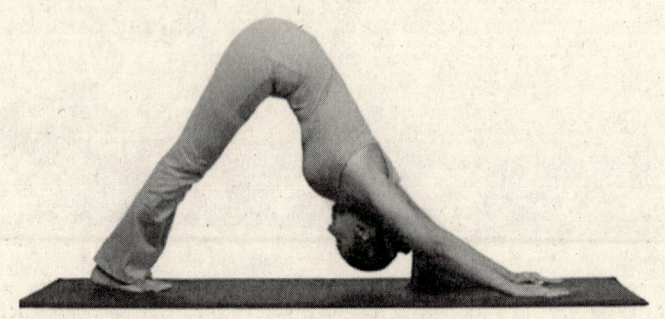

Exhale and raise your hips upwards, pushing the upper body behind and touching your heels to the floor while keeping the knees straight and face downwards, looking at the navel region. Once in posture, breathe normally.

i.   Position: **Ashwa Sanchalanasana**

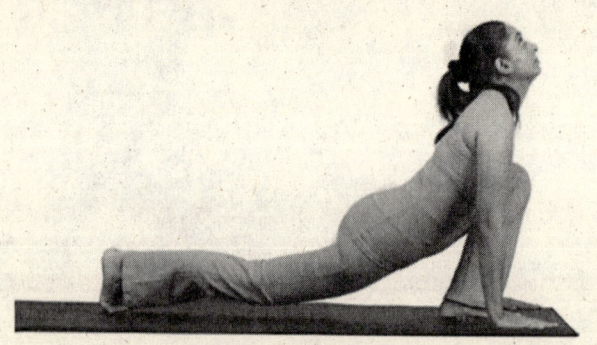

Inhale while bringing the left leg forward between your hands, arch your back and keep your chin upwards, while your palms are flat on the floor. Once in the posture, breathe normally.

j. Position: **Padahastasana**

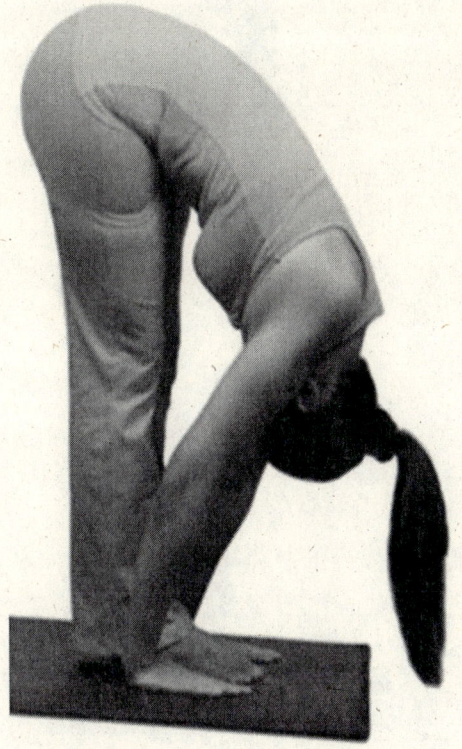

Exhale while bringing your right leg forward. Knees should be straight and palms touching the toe and neck relaxed. Once in the posture, breathe normally.

k.   Position: **Chakarasana**

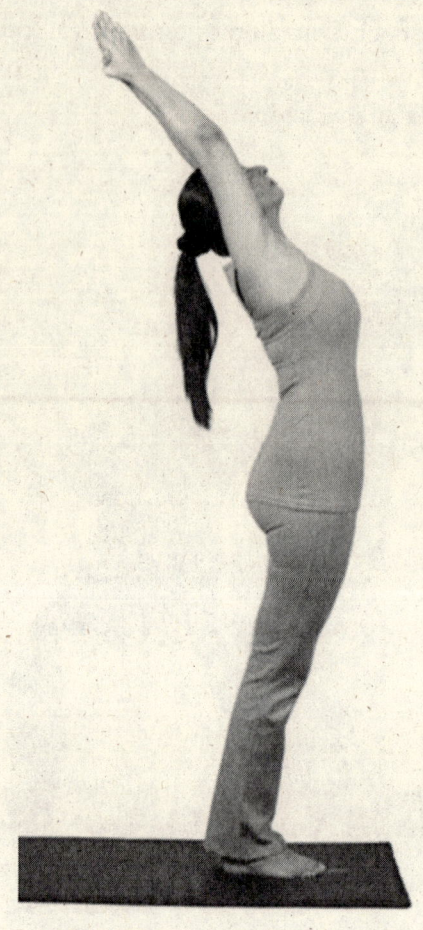

Put your palms together, inhale and raise your hands and the upper body upwards, arching the back. Once in the posture, breathe normally.

1. Position: **Namaskar Mudra**

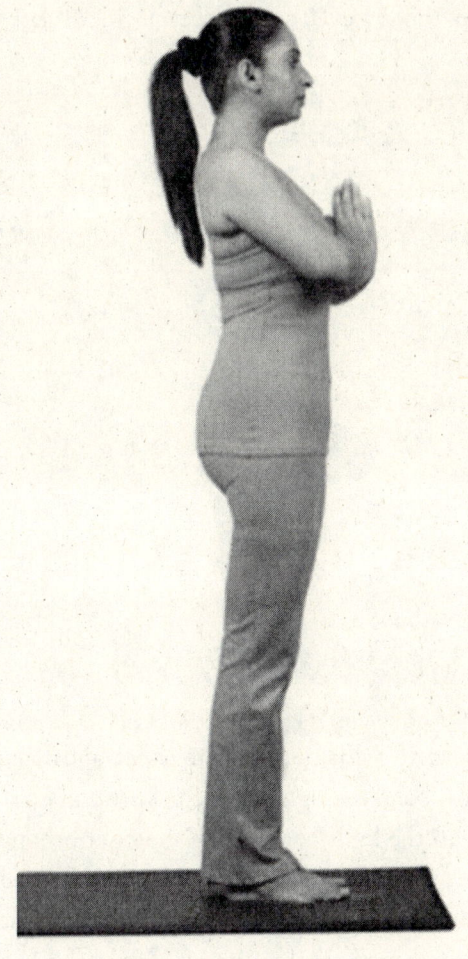

Slowly, while exhaling, come back to the starting position.

STANDING POSITIONS

Vrikshasana (hold for 10 seconds, each side, 1 set)

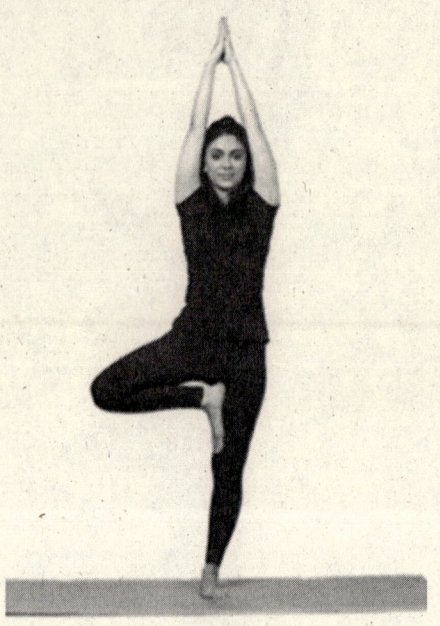

Stand straight with both feet together and hands by the side. Now bend the right leg at the knee and hold the right ankle with the right hand. Place the right heel tight at the pelvic region, while balancing the body on the left leg. Then raise your hands up and form the Namaskar Mudra with palms together, above your head. Balance this asana for some time, breathing normally. Come back slowly to the original position and repeat the same with the other leg.

Benefits: Strengthens the thigh and calf muscles and improves mind and body coordination.

Tadasana (hold for 10 seconds, 1 set; see p. 17)

Trikonasana (hold for 10 seconds, each side, 1 set)

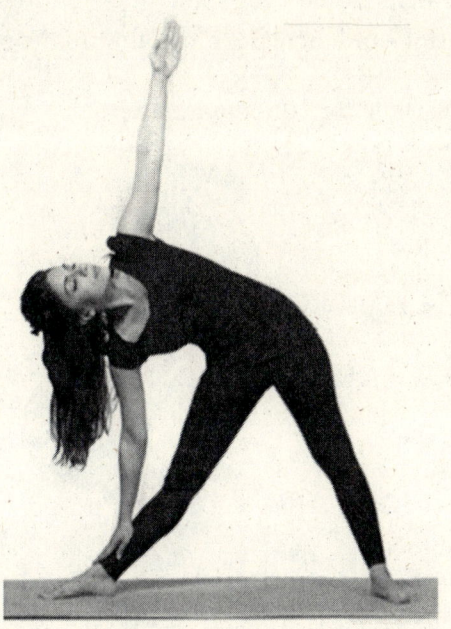

Stand straight with your legs together and hands by the sides of the thighs. Spread your legs apart slowly up to a distance of 2 to 3 feet. Slowly raise both the hands sideways at shoulder level with the palms facing the floor. Turn your right toes out while exhaling, then bend forward towards the right side, touching the big toe of the right leg with the left hand without bending the knees. Raise your right hand up and look up towards it, breathing normally. Hold this pose for some time and come back to the original position. Repeat the same with the other side.

Benefits: Makes the spine flexible, strengthens the hamstrings and increases blood flow to the upper body.

Utkatasana (hold for 10 seconds, 1 set)

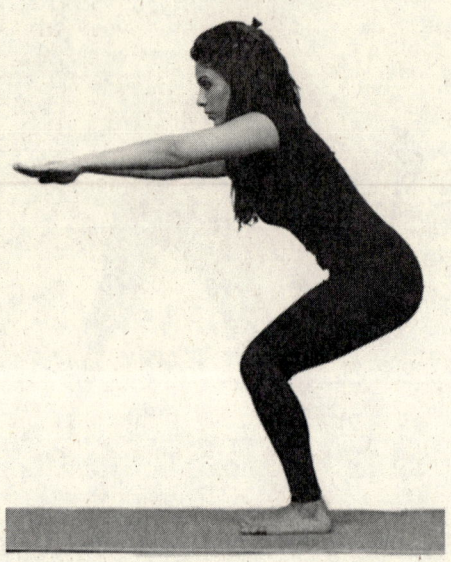

Stand straight, feet together, palms by the side of the body. Keep your feet apart, almost as much as the width of your shoulders. Now bend your knees at 90 degrees to the floor and slowly raise your hands in front of you to shoulder level. Stay in this posture for some time and breathe normally. Slowly come back to the starting position.

Benefits: Strengthens and tones calves and thighs.

SITTING POSITIONS

Supta Vajrasana (hold for 10 seconds, 1 set)

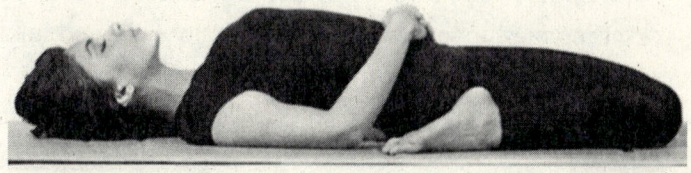

Sit straight in Vajrasana. Keep your feet apart on the floor. Lean backwards on your right and left elbows. Now try and bend your head and back towards the floor as much as you can till you are comfortable while stretching the abdomen. Keeping the hands on the stomach, hold for some time, breathing normally. Now with the help of the elbows slowly come back to the original position.

Benefits: Strengthens the thigh and calf muscles and aids good digestion.

Parvatasana in Padmasana (hold for 10 seconds, 1 set)

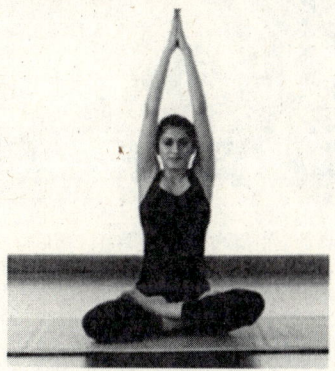

Sit straight in Padmasana with palms resting on the floor. Get the palms together, facing each other, in Namaskar Mudra close to the chest. Inhale slowly and raise your hands upwards and stretch your arms as much as you can without exerting pressure on the neck. Breathe normally and hold for some time. Slowly come back to the original position.

Benefits: Makes the upper back and shoulders flexible.

Janushirshasana (hold for 10 seconds, each side, 1 set; see p. 19)

Vakrasana (hold for 10 seconds, each side, 1 set)

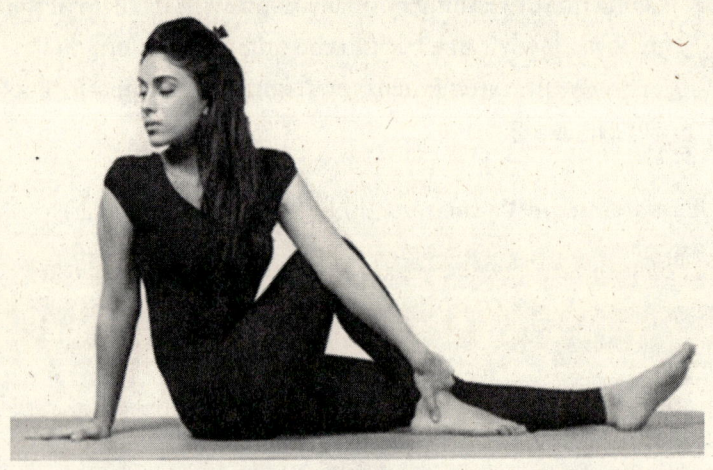

Sit straight on the floor, stretching the legs in front, hands by the side, and palms resting on the floor. Now slowly bend the right leg at the knee and place your right foot close to the left knee joint. With the right knee facing upwards, rest the palm of your right hand flat on the floor near your spine. Then take the left hand over the right knee and try to grasp the right ankle, while twisting the head back towards the right side, and looking backwards. Breathing normally, hold for some time, and come back to the original position. Repeat the same with the other side.

Benefits: Reduces stiffness in the back and massages the internal organs, reducing the fat from the abdomen area.

Gomukhasana (hold for 10 seconds, each side, 1 set)

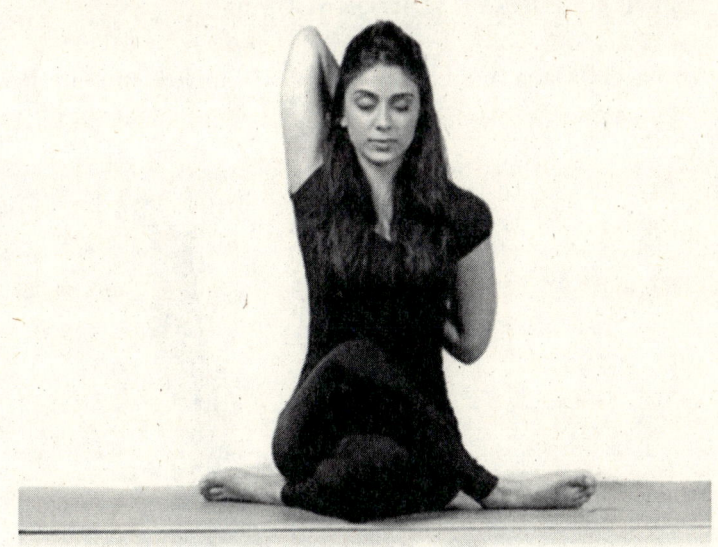

Sit on the floor, stretching your legs forward. Bend both your knees slightly. Place your left leg under your right thigh and take your right leg over your left leg, making sure your knees are on top of each other. Now take your right hand, with the elbow facing the ceiling, behind your back with your fingers facing downwards. Now take your left hand behind your back. Try holding both your palms together, making sure your entire back is straight and aligned with your neck. Breathe normally once you are in this posture. Repeat the same with the other leg and hand. Hold for some time and come back to the original position.

Benefits: Strengthens and tones your arms, legs and back.

SUPINE POSITIONS (LYING ON YOUR BACK)

Ardha-Halasana (hold for 10 seconds, 10 movements, 1 set)

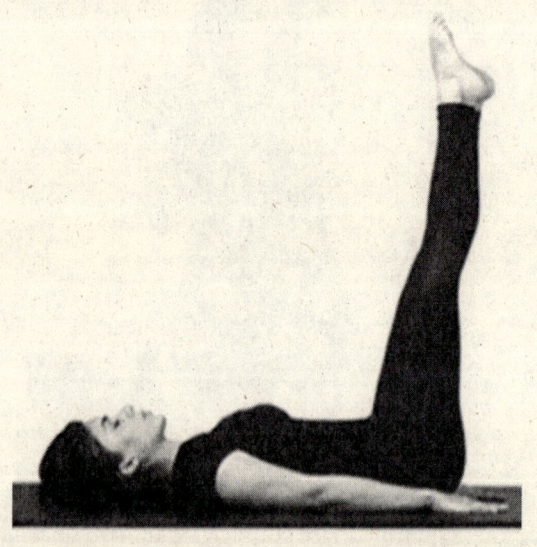

Lie in a supine position with legs together, hands by the side of the body, palms resting on the floor. Now while exhaling, raise both legs together gradually up to 30-, 45-, 60- and 90-degree angles. Hold each angle for 10 counts, with normal breathing, then slowly inhale and come down from 90- to 60-, 45- and 30-degree angles respectively.

Benefits: Strengthens the abdominal muscles, burns fat in the thighs, hips and abdomen.

Pawanmukthasana (hold for 10 seconds, 10 movements, 1 set; see p. 22)

Setubandhasana (hold for 10 seconds, 10 movements, 1 set)

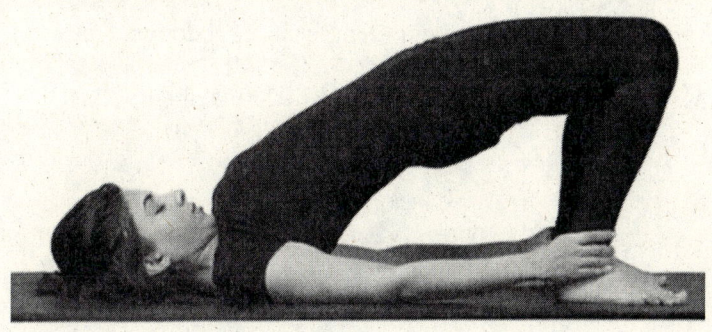

Lie on your back, and bend your knees. Keep your feet close to your hips with hands by the side, and palms resting on the floor. Inhale slowly and push the waist upwards as much as you can without any pressure on your neck. Hold for some time while breathing normally.

Benefits: Strengthens the shoulders and thigh muscles.

Naukasana (hold for 10 seconds, 10 movements, 1 set)

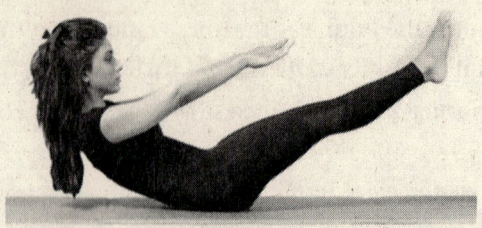

Lie down on your back with your feet together and your palms resting on your thighs. Inhale and raise both legs up, then raise the upper body off the floor. Hold for some time while breathing normally, raising your hands and stretching them so they are parallel to the floor. Return to the original position slowly.

Benefits: Tones and strengthens the abdominal muscles.

Vipreetkarni (hold for 10 seconds, 10 movements, 1 set)

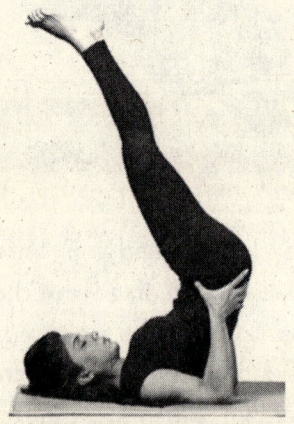

Lie down on your back and put your feet together and hands by the sides with the palms resting on the floor.

Now inhale slowly and raise both your legs up, 90 degrees to the floor. Then push your palms on the floor and raise your hips up. Hold your waist with your hands in the final position. Remember to keep your neck muscles relaxed and breathe normally. Stay in this position for 15 to 20 seconds, then come back slowly to the original position in a reverse manner. Follow it up with its counter-pose, Setubandhasana.

Benefits: Directs and enhances the blood flow towards the head.

PRONE POSITIONS (ON THE STOMACH)

Niralambasana (hold for 10 seconds, 1 set)

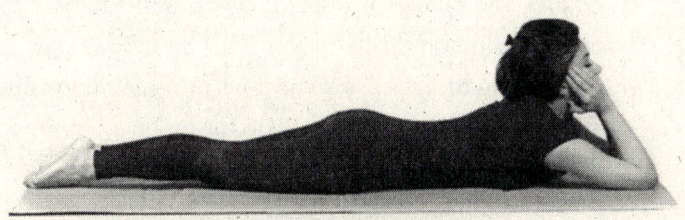

Lie in a prone position with your forehead on the floor, hands by the side, legs together, and toes pointed outwards. Slowly stretch the arms forward, and bend the elbows, raising the head upwards. Place the chin on the open palms facing upwards, with your fingers touching your cheeks. Make sure the elbows are together. Hold this pose for some time, breathing normally. Then slowly come back to the original position.

Benefits: Relaxes the neck muscles.

Bhunjangasana (hold for 10 seconds, 1 set)

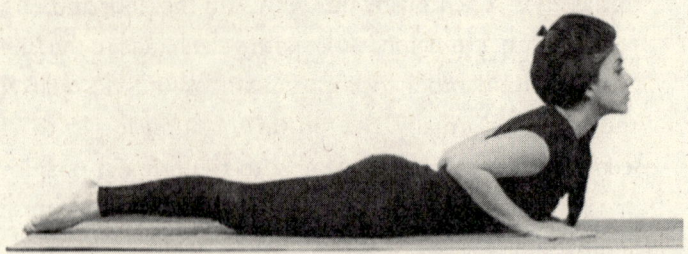

Lie in a prone position, legs together, toes together and pointing outwards, hands by the side of the body, palms facing upwards, and forehead on the floor. Now bend hands from the elbows, place the palms on the floor near each side of the shoulder. The thumb should be under the armpit. Inhale and raise your chin, turn your head upwards as much as possible, and raise your upper body up to the navel. Try to keep the palms off the floor by tucking the elbows close to the body. Hold this pose for some time, breathing normally. Then, while exhaling, come down to the original position.

Benefits: Improves spinal flexibility.

Shalabhasana (hold for 10 seconds, 1 set)

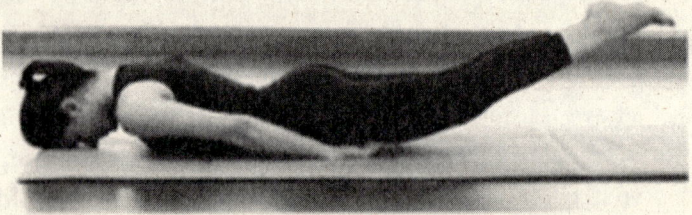

Lie in the prone position, bring the legs together, toes pointing outwards, hands by the side of the body, fists closed, and forehead on the floor. Then raise both the legs slowly without bending at the knee, keeping the fists beneath the thighs. Do not tilt the pelvis. Hold this pose for some time, breathing normally, and come back down slowly.

Benefits: Beneficial for people with flatulence and gastric problems, hypertension and lumber pain.

BREATHING

Kapalbhati Kriya (for cleansing; 25 strokes, 4 rounds)

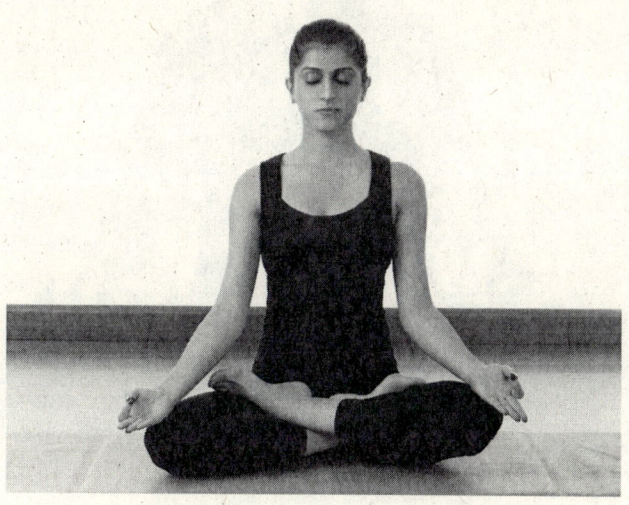

Sit comfortably in Padmasana. Rest your hands on your knees or lower belly. Breathe normally for some time. In a quick motion, contract your abdominal muscles and forcefully exhale from your nose all the air from your lungs. Allow your lungs to fill without effort. Repeat this cycle and then allow your breath to return to normal.

Benefits: Balances and strengthens the nervous system, cleansing the respiratory track.

Deep Breathing (5 rounds)

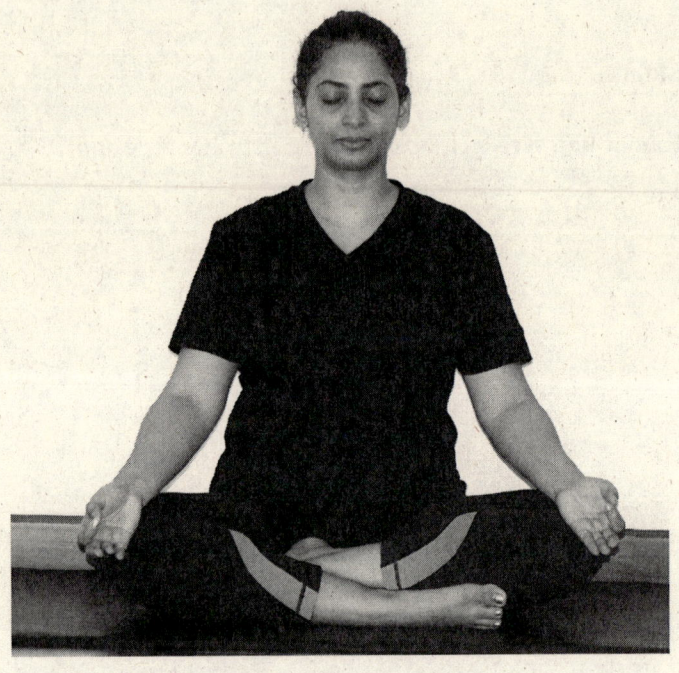

Sit straight in any comfortable meditative posture. Inhale deeply counting up to 5 and without holding your breath, exhale slowly to 10 counts. Relax for few seconds and repeat.

Brahma Mudra (3 rounds)

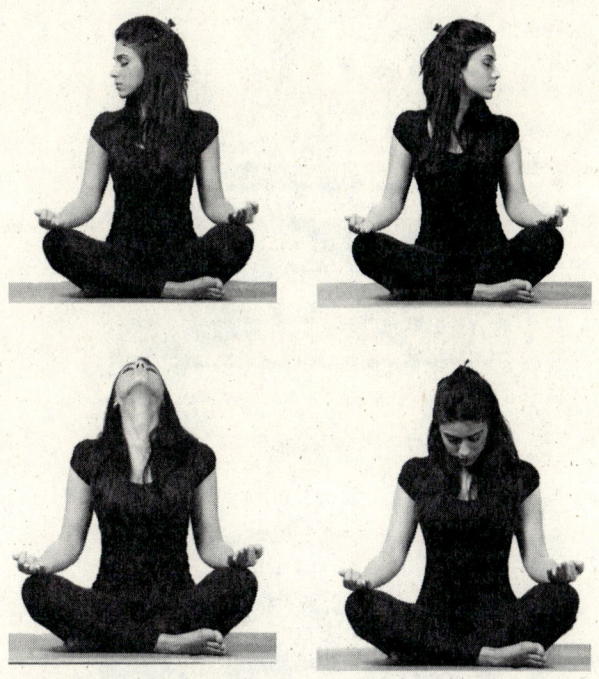

Sit straight in any comfortable meditative posture in Gyan
Mudra (index finger touching the tip of thumb). Now
slowly turn your neck towards the right side and hold for
5 seconds, then repeat the process with the other side and
hold again for 5 seconds. Now bring your neck back to the
original position and raise your chin up. Hold it there for
5 seconds, then slowly bring your neck down and hold it
there for 5 seconds and come back to the original position.

Benefits: Removes stiffness from the neck.

Anulom Vilom Pranayam (5 rounds)

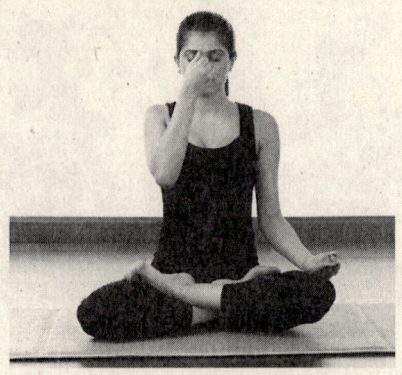

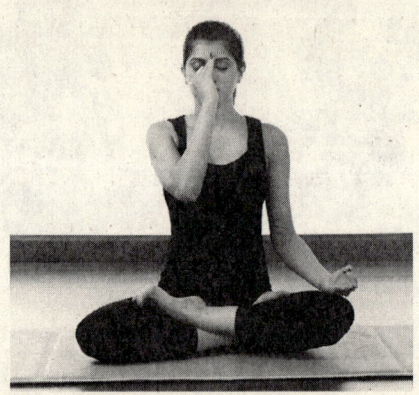

Sit straight in any comfortable meditative posture. Use the thumb of your right hand to close your right nostril and inhale through your left nostril. Then close your left nostril with your right hand's index and middle fingers and exhale from the right nostril. Now, in a reverse manner, inhale with the right nostril, close your right nostril with your right hand's thumb then exhale with the left. This forms one round of Anulom Vilom Pranayam.

Benefits: Purifies 72,000 nerves (nadis) in the body and balances body temperature.

Ujjayi Pranayam (3 rounds, one way, exhale)

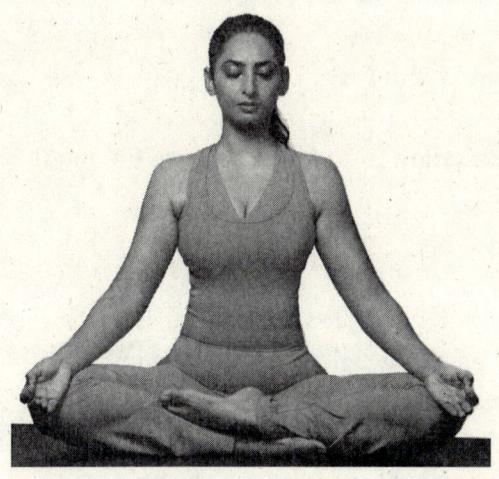

Sit straight in any meditative or comfortable posture. Now inhale slowly and deeply through the nose and while exhaling, contract the air passage and exhale slowly with a whispering sound.

Benefits: Balances hormones and improves concentration.

Sheetali Pranayam (3 rounds)

Sit straight in any meditative or comfortable position. Close your eyes and relax your whole body with normal breathing. Put the tongue on the lower lip and try to roll the tongue. Inhale deeply through the mouth and slowly close the mouth and exhale through the nose. This is one round of Sheetali Pranayam.

Benefits: Provides a cooling effect to the body.

Om Chanting (3 rounds)

Relaxation (5 minutes)

Basic Meditation (sit calm and quiet, 2 minutes)

Yin Yang Yoga

Yin Yang yoga, also called couple yoga, is the balancing of the male and female energies between a couple. Also called Shiv Shakti (male and female energies), Yin Yang yoga is mainly directed towards busy couples who want to spend quality time with each other.

All the asanas in Yin Yang yoga are to be done with your spouse. When couples perform the exercises in this type of yoga they feel the love and passion flowing towards each other, all coming into balance. Both partners do the same posture simultaneously, balancing and counter-balancing to co-create the posture. While performing the asanas, partners help each other by supporting one another, which is important in a relationship. The challenges they face when doing the asanas can bring about a realization of each other's internal and emotional conflicts. This balance pervades not just your body but even your mind. Because Yin Yang yoga involves physical asanas, the sense of touch, conscious breathing, humour and light-heartedness, all come into play.

Working with a partner helps you to open your body more deeply than you could alone. Relying on each other's support to keep correct body alignment, balance and concentration helps couples to loosen up, especially if they are yet to be married. These exercises give the participants the opportunity to be creative in their yoga practice and boost their compassion for one another and bonding. It also enhances intimacy in relationships.

The first thing you will notice once you start practising this form of yoga is that it's not just about exercising, it's about learning to communicate, how to read each other's energy and how to be supportive of one another, physically and mentally.

When a couple enters a Yin Yang class they should be free of any negative energy. The mind should be like an empty box as this would help them focus and improve their concentration and awareness of themselves as well as their partner. In some cases, this is difficult as the mind is always working and when one is in a silent, calm and composed posture, the mind is flooded with things like pending duties, things that have happened through the day and so on. Therefore, it is impossible to just get into a class and expect to meditate or get into a calm posture straight away. At Cosmic Fusion, we recommend soft lighting with aromatic candles, romantic music which helps boost the mood while doing Yin Yang yoga with your partner, as it creates a calming, de-stressing ambience. This time is used to relax, talk about experiences, share a bond and erase differences.

POSTURES

Vrikshasana

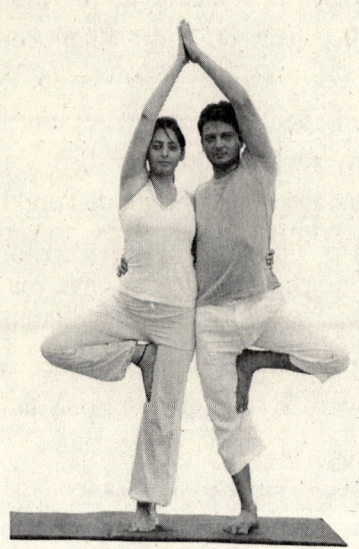

Stand straight with both feet together and hands by the side. Now one partner should bend the right leg at the knee, the other to bend the left leg at the knee and each to hold their ankles with the other hand. Place the heel right at the pelvic region while helping each other keep balance. Holding each other around the waist, raise the other hand above the head and join your palms together, breathing normally. Slowly come back to the original position.

Benefits: Strengthens thighs and calf muscles. Improves mind and body coordination and the couple is encouraged to give each other support.

Samtulasana

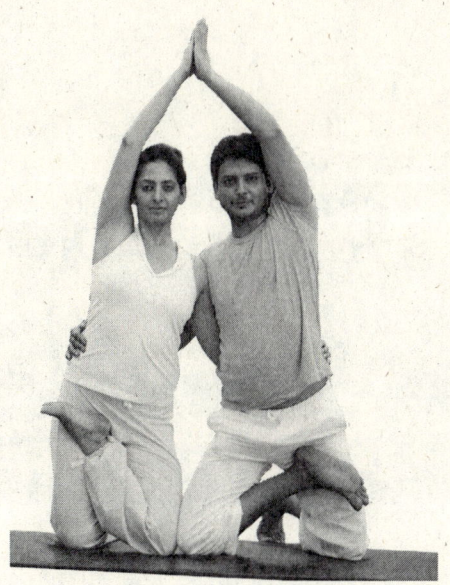

Stand straight with both hands by the side of the body. Then slowly kneel down beside each other. Then sit on your heels. One partner should now place the right foot on his/her left thigh and the other partner should place the left foot on his/her right thigh. Then, with each other's support, slowly come up on your knees. Then raise your opposite hands up to join your palms together, taking the other hand behind each other, supporting your partner. Hold it for as long as you can and repeat with the other leg. Keep breathing normally while in this posture.

Benefits: Increases flexibility and support for each other, mentally and physically.

Parigrahasana

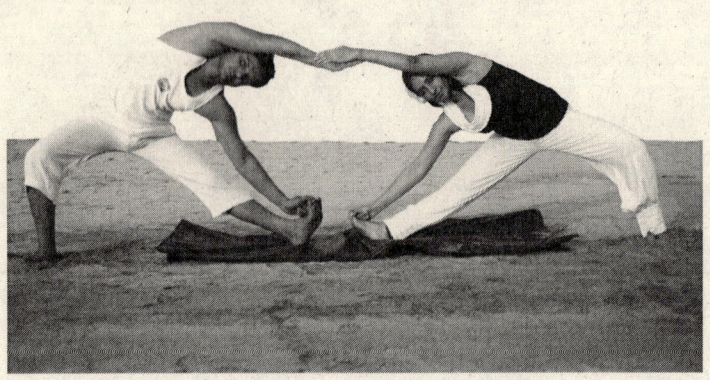

Stand beside each other. Spread and stretch your legs as much as you can. Now one partner should bend at the left knee and the other at the right knee in such a way that you both are facing each other. Now touch the toe of the other leg with the same hand. Use your other hand to hold on to your partner. Hold this pose for some time. Repeat the same with the other side.

Benefits: Stretches the pelvic region and the groin muscles. It also burns fat from the sides of the hips or what we commonly refer to as 'love handles'.

Virabhadrasana

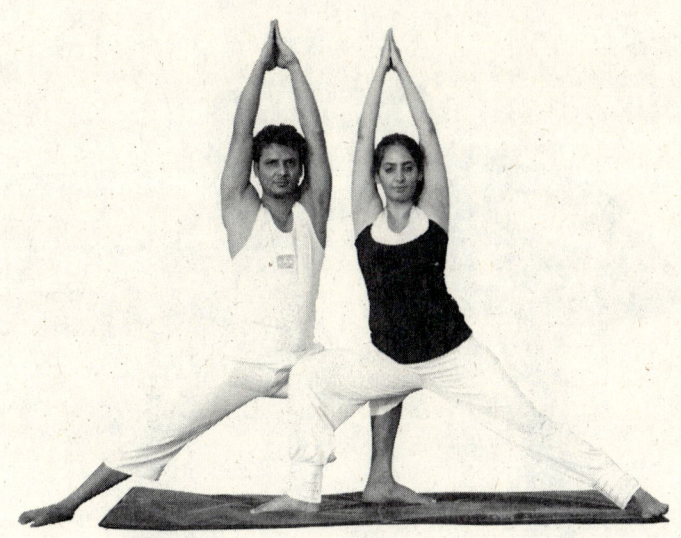

Stand straight with your feet shoulder-width apart and your hands by the side of your body. Now spread your legs to 3–4 feet. Spread your arms sideways at shoulder level, one partner bending to the left and the other to the right. Bend your knee to form a right angle from the floor and raise your arms to join your palms together. Once in the posture, breathe normally.

Benefits: It strengthens the lower body and gives the couple a sense of belonging and togetherness.

Couple Natrajasana

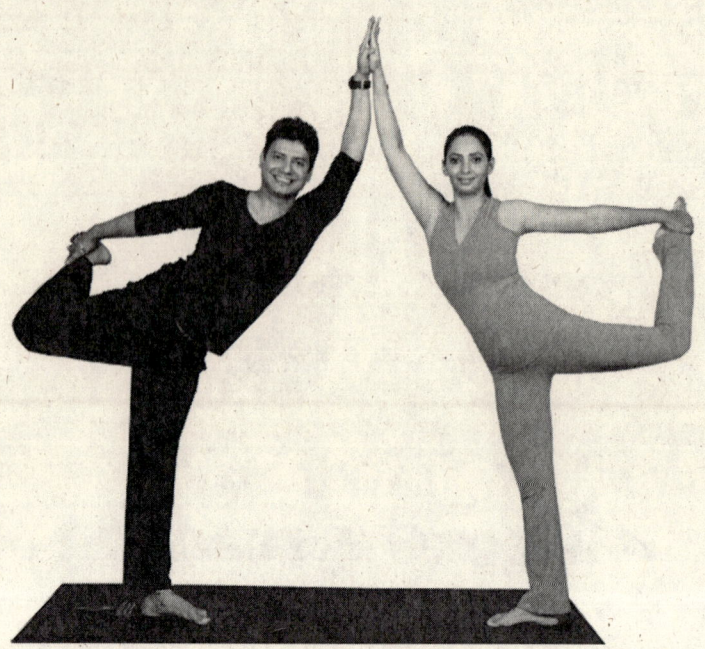

Stand straight with your feet together and hands by the side of your body. Now, while supporting each other, one partner to raise their left hand and the other to raise their right hand and get their palms together. Now with the help of each other, hold the ankle of the leg opposite the hands you have raised, by bending it at the knee. Now, while slowly inhaling, raise the leg as high as you can away from the buttocks. Support each other's balance. Once you are in this posture, breath normally and then slowly come back to the original position.

Benefits: This improves the flexibility of the back, spinal cord, quadriceps and shoulders.

Common Worries

Once I start trying to get pregnant, could I become pregnant on the very first day that I have had sex?

If you have had unprotected sex, then yes, you could get pregnant. If you don't, there's no need to worry. Give your body time and avoid stress, as that plays a big role in inhibiting conception.

My friend told me that if I have sex during my period I can't get pregnant. Is that true?

Chances of conception from sex during periods is more of a theoretical possibility, practically nil.

I tried to calculate my period and had sex according to the 14th day of my cycle. Can I get pregnant?

Well, as I mentioned earlier, it totally depends on your cycle. In accordance with the duration of your cycles, short or long, the ovulation days differ. That doesn't mean you cannot become pregnant by having unprotected sex on non-ovulating days because the sperm, once inside, could survive for days. Fertility is high on the day of ovulation and a day before that, 12 to 16 days before you start your next period. If you have a short cycle like say 20 days you could ovulate before the 14th day. If you have a long cycle, like say 35 days, then your ovulation day would be on day 20. This ovulation calculation is totally dependent on your cycle and could differ from woman to woman. Those who have a strict 28-day cycle could ovulate on the 14th day.

2

First Trimester

Having a baby is one of the most exciting times in a woman's life. Since you've come to this part of the book I can happily say, congratulations, you gorgeous woman!

You can say goodbye to spontaneous drink plans and late night parties for some time now. You can stop thinking about all those failed pregnancy strips and all those ovulation kits you saved. Sit back and laugh at all the calculated menstrual cycles you so dedicatedly kept track of.

I bet you are flooded with all the thoughts of how you're going to surprise your husband, your parents, your in-laws and friends. How this time makes you feel on top of the world! You want to shout with joy! Enjoy this time with your husband and make the most of it as, from experience, nine months from now, you are not going to have much time for each other and life is going to change drastically.

Your body is going through so many changes that it could affect your mood at the drop of a hat; you might just get upset and anxious for no reason but that's all right. You will be flooded with thoughts of whether you will be a good mother, whether you are eating right or is there anything you are doing wrong that is going to affect the baby. Like my mother always told me during my pregnancy: Beta, just relax. Everything will be fine! No child comes into this world with a manual and each child is different and so is each pregnancy. No matter how many books you read or how many videos you watch, you will never be prepared for what's coming your way, trust me.

Pregnancy is divided into three trimesters, roughly approximating specific developmental stages. The first 12 weeks of pregnancy form the first trimester. This is the time when your body is going through some crazy drastic changes, internally as well as externally.

When I was pregnant, a friend of mine was pregnant too. She got to know a week after me. Even though we had the same body structure, ate similar diets, both fitness freaks with almost the same lifestyles, both of us had extreme pregnancies. Where I had the most amazing time from the day I got to know I was pregnant, hers was a roller-coaster ride. I'll start by telling you about my experience.

On your first appointment with your doctor, a whole list of information is gathered—your lifestyle, diet habits, medical history and so on. It is very important to mention any previous pregnancies, abortions and medical family history. Then, the doctor weighs you, takes your blood pressure, and draws blood for any health issues like diabetes, thyroid, confirms your pregnancy through a blood test and makes your BMI chart depending on the above measurements.

The doctor advises you on how to take care of yourself during your pregnancy with good eating habits and safe exercises, keeping in mind that you would need to cut back on any strenuous workout and take a lax initially. The doctor may also prescribe pregnancy-safe medication that would help you during and after pregnancy like Vitamin D and folic acid. I didn't experience any nausea and morning sickness. My doctor advised me to follow only one thing and it was to not brush my teeth in the morning. I used to feel uneasy due to the menthol in my toothpaste after brushing my teeth in the morning, so my doctor suggested that I brush my teeth after breakfast.

The first sonography scan is at 6 weeks. It is the first scan when you can hear the heartbeat of the baby.

The second scan—Nuchal Translucency—is at 11–12 weeks. The third scan—Anomaly—is at 18–19 weeks. The fourth scan—4-D sonography—at 26–27 weeks is optional. The fifth scan is at 36 weeks to confirm the growth of the baby.

My friend Sonal, whom I mentioned earlier, had a tough time during the first trimester. She was struck with extreme nausea, exhaustion, extremely sore breasts, constipation, extreme bouts of morning sickness. Anything she would eat or drink, even if it was a sandwich, would make her sick. Any kind of smells would instantly put her off. The smell of food that was being prepared in the kitchen would drive her insane and would trigger nausea, due to which she was constantly exhausted and tired. Her doctor advised her to eat two biscuits on waking up even before brushing her teeth, as even trying to brush her teeth in the morning would result in vomiting. This usually happens when the stomach is empty through the night due to which the acids in the stomach come up. In her case she was even getting dehydrated as she couldn't drink water as even water was making her sick, causing weakness and the constant feeling of tiredness.

The causes of nausea and tummy issues during this time are the increased levels of oestrogen during the first trimester. Oestrogen levels fluctuate, causing an imbalance in the brain that triggers nausea and vomiting. The hormone called progesterone makes food longer and harder to digest, and so women suffer from stomach issues. In Sonal's case, she experienced severe constipation due to indigestion. It is always better to inform your doctor about such issues as a pregnant woman needs to be extra cautious in taking any over-the-counter medication as it could cause problems for the pregnancy. It tends to settle after 13 to 14 weeks in most cases. The reason for Sonal's breast tenderness, sore nipples and swelling were due to the hormones that were undergoing the process of preparing the breast to produce milk.

During pregnancy, a woman's breasts grow throughout the whole nine months but the pain and soreness gradually subside. I know how most women love their fancy lacy or push-up bras. Now is the time to put them right at the back of your closet, only to be brought out once your pregnancy and nursing days are over. You need to now invest in comfortable, soft fabric and stretch material bras, giving your breasts all the space and comfort to grow without putting them through any discomfort. Underwire bras are a no-go. They just dig into your tender breasts causing more discomfort and pain. Busty women can go for bras with thicker straps as they provide more support and comfort. For sleep time, pregnancy sleeping bras are available if you particularly want to go looking for them. For those who aren't able to source them out, you could use comfortable snug size sports bras or a tank top with a camisole inner which could save you a lot of money.

Important Signs

For those who experience symptoms like my friend, Sonal, I suggest you always keep your gynaecologist informed as some cases can get severe and lead to further complications. Some of these symptoms may be:

1. Those who aren't able to keep any food or liquid down for 20 hours may suffer from dehydration, which can be very dangerous for the mother and baby.
2. Women tend to pee a lot during pregnancy. Always keep track of the amount you pee as not urinating for long intervals could be a sign your body is trying to tell you something is wrong.
3. Some women experience spotting during pregnancy which your doctor should be informed about as it is common in some cases due to various factors, such as a cervical polyp (harmless growth on the cervix) coming in contact with this area during intercourse, which could cause spotting. In any case, a woman needs to contact

her doctor as it could also be a case of miscarriage, which is very common during the first trimester. Sometimes spotting can occur when the embryo attaches itself to the walls, eroding a few small blood vessels of the uterus which is a common problem but still needs to be looked at and confirmed by your doctor. There are also times in the initial weeks of pregnancy where strenuous activities such as heavy lifting or overworking could lead to bleeding. Women are advised against sexual intercourse during the initial period of pregnancy as this could lead to bleeding. For those who experience any of the above problems, the doctor advises bed rest with minimal mobility.

4. Any pain or discomfort in the lower abdomen accompanied with pressure and strong pulling pains in the pelvic region following up with spotting or bleeding is a bad sign. If this happens, a woman needs to be taken into the emergency room right away.

5. Those who suffer from tummy issues every now and then could contact their doctor for some remedies, whereas, those who are constipated for long durations need to be checked by their doctor ASAP. Stool softeners or laxatives are prescribed. Do not ever self-medicate during your pregnancy as anything you eat could have an adverse effect on your baby.

Changes One Can Expect

This is the stage where a woman's body has accepted the baby and is in the process of helping it grow. The first trimester begins on the first day of your last period, which is then carried on until the 12th week of pregnancy. This is the way a doctor determines the baby's growth and the due date, which in some cases changes due to the baby's development. Hormonal changes play a huge role in many of the symptoms women face during pregnancy, which affect their physical and mental state. Some of the changes which can be expected are:

1. Breast tenderness
2. Constipation/gas/bloating
3. Vaginal discharge: Also called leucorrhoea, this is a milky white discharge. Panty liners are recommended, as due to the discharge the panty gets wet and friction along with moisture causes irritation on the inner thighs and rashes. These panty liners need to be changed frequently to keep unwanted germs away. Doctors are against the use of tampons during this time as a build-up of germs is seen in the vagina with the use of tampons. (If there is a change in the colour of your discharge, like turning to green, yellow, or there is a lot of clear discharge, it is advised to inform your doctor.)
4. Fatigue: This happens because your body is making a living being and going through structural changes to accommodate your baby. While your body is undergoing these changes, it is constantly at work, which in turn is exhausting. Therefore, it is advised to take it slow during this time with mid-day naps every now and then.
5. Food cravings: Some women have the weirdest of cravings like ice cream with raw mango, while some not at all. The cravings vary from crazy timings and specific foods to something known as 'Pica', which means cravings that

consist of non-foods like clay, dirt, starch, soap. It may sound weird but it is true. These cravings might sound odd but they are definitely dangerous to both mother and child. Please contact your doctor immediately.

6. Frequent urination: This happens because of the growing uterus pressing against the bladder which leads to the urge to pee. Do not ever hold your urine, even if it is during the night. Do not stop yourself or cut down on liquids because it is waking you during the night. Sometimes due to extreme nausea, some women aren't able to have the required intake of water, which can affect the system, resulting in UTIs (urinary tract infections) and other issues, so it is always best to keep yourself hydrated at all times. Avoid too much salt and sugar. If you aren't able to drink water, the doctor usually advises flavoured water and juices, but always opt for healthy choices like fresh juices and fruits and vegetables over canned or tetrapack options.

7. Heartburn: This is experienced by almost all pregnant women at some point in their pregnancy. To avoid this, eat smaller and more frequent meals. Do not directly lie down or sleep after eating; sit up or walk about, as it would help in the digestion process. Avoid eating oily, spicy, acidic foods, citrus fruits or caffeine as this aggravates the problem. Keep a gap between your meals and bedtime giving enough time for your food to digest before going to bed.

Initially, many women don't even realize they are pregnant. The symptoms are not very visible for the first few weeks, and they can be confused for other things. Let me share with you the story of my friend.

It all started out when she went on a vacation with her husband to the Maldives. They wanted to take this holiday as the couple had been wanting to start trying to have a baby since they had been married for four years. She didn't have any medical conditions but she was 43 years old and her periods were irregular (delayed/early by a few days or just spotting), but her doctor said that it was because of her age, work stress and hectic lifestyle. There was nothing to be alarmed about. They saw the best doctor and took second opinions but all the tests came out clear and all the doctors had the same answer: nothing was wrong with either one of them; they just had to give themselves time. Her husband worked in the stock market, so time was very important to him and the work stress didn't get any easier with every passing year. It was the family who suggested the vacation and so it happened.

My friend owns an advertising company so she was always on her toes and her career was her baby till then. It was one of the days during their holiday that her husband noticed his wife had an exceptional glow and looked happier, but she shrugged it off saying it was the sun, fresh exotic fruits and relaxation that was making the difference. During the holiday, her husband surprised her with a candle-lit dinner on the beach. The next day she woke up complaining of an upset tummy and vomiting, which she thought was because of previous night's food. Thereafter she realized she was constantly tired, but dismissed it as anxiety of getting back to the routine after a satisfying holiday.

They returned from their holiday and she was still feeling tired and moody all the time. The only thing that made her happy was food. They decided to visit their doctor who asked her to do a home pregnancy test as well as other tests. After their long excruciating wait, where half an hour seemed like an entire day, they were congratulated on the arrival of her test results: she was pregnant and was 8 weeks along.

In her case, she experienced spotting which she took as a light period and skipped all of the symptoms, thinking it was a stomach bug. There are some women who experience a heavy bout of symptoms whereas a few do not experience them at all in the first trimester.

During this time, the body goes through many changes, and the organs in the human body are affected due to the hormonal changes. The most evident sign of a woman who might be pregnant is the absence of a monthly period. Some of the early symptoms are:

- Nausea
- Weight loss or gain
- Tiredness
- Mood swings
- Frequent urination
- Headache
- Constipation
- Tender breasts

- Upset tummy/morning sickness
- Cravings or distaste for certain foods
- Heartburn
- Dizziness and fatigue

During the first trimester, it is very important for you to take all precautions as a miscarriage is very common during this time. This is the time where a woman would need to make lifestyle changes like quitting smoking, drinking, junk foods, artificially flavoured drinks (see box below).

Dos and Don'ts during the First Trimester

1. Avoid drinking alcohol.
2. Avoid smoking.
3. Do not drink too much of caffeine: 2 cups of coffee a day are enough. Do not overdo it.
4. Avoid drinking aerated drinks like soda and artificial sweetened drinks.
5. Try to eat home-cooked food and avoid junk food.
6. Consult your doctor before taking any kind of medication.
7. Skip those extra high heels if you are not comfortable in them.
8. Keep away from harsh cleaning materials like acids as the fumes could be dangerous for the baby.

Some women are afraid because they've done the opposite of what they needed to do, but there is no need to worry as this is the initial time of your pregnancy where the embryo is forming and this would not have affected the baby. You now need to make these lifestyle changes as the body would be soaking up the nutrients that are used to develop the baby.

Pregnancy: Week by Week

Week 4: Congrats! You are now confirmed as pregnant. The baby is smaller than a mustard seed, maybe exactly the size of a poppy seed. During this time your baby is settling in the uterus.

Week 5: The foetus has started taking shape and developing organs, eyes, nose and so on. The baby's size is that of an apple seed. (0.4/0.7 millimetres)

Week 6: The baby now has blood circulation. The baby's size is 5–6 mm. It looks like a pea. (2.5 millimetres)

Week 7: During this time the baby's brain is forming and developing at a rapid rate. The baby is the size of a blueberry. (0.51 inches)

Week 8: The baby is able to wiggle its arms and legs but the mother won't be able to feel it so soon. The baby would have doubled in size and is now as big as a raspberry. (0.84 inches)

Week 9: At this stage, the doctors should be able to pick up a heartbeat with a Doppler. The baby is as big as an olive or even a strawberry. (1.1 inches)

Week 10: The baby is able to move its arms as the joints are formed and working. The joints in the arms develop faster than the legs. Your uterus is the size of a tennis ball. The baby is as big as a date or even a plum (1.2 inches).

Week 11: At the end of the first trimester, the baby is more developed. The hands and feet do not look webbed any more. A little bump can be seen only after it becomes an abdominal organ, that is after 12 weeks+ time. The baby is now the size of a sour lime (1.6 inches).

Week 12: The baby has now taken full shape. At this time its sex organs can be seen sonographically. A healthy, developed baby would now have its limbs, organs, muscles. The heartbeat is heard on Doppler in the clinic at 12 weeks+.

Yoga for the First Trimester

Before beginning the workout, prepare in the following manner:

The place: Choose a place which has fresh and well-circulated air, preferably a garden, a terrace, or a workout place in your house. If you want, place some flower pots in the room to boost your mood. This room needs to be well-ventilated.

The requirements: A yoga mat, a bottle of water, a hand or face towel. You can play some slow music in the background if you like.

To start: Spread the mat on the floor and sit in a comfortable position. Take five to ten long breaths to relax yourself. Stretch your hands and legs to loosen the muscles. Perform the warm-up exercises mentioned in Chapter 1 (p. 14), without putting any undue stress on your body.

Kati Chakrasana Crocodile Series: 6 variations (hold for 10 seconds each side, 1 set)

Benefits: It strengthens the back, waist, abdomen and pelvic muscles and makes them flexible

Kati Chakrasana Crocodile Series 1

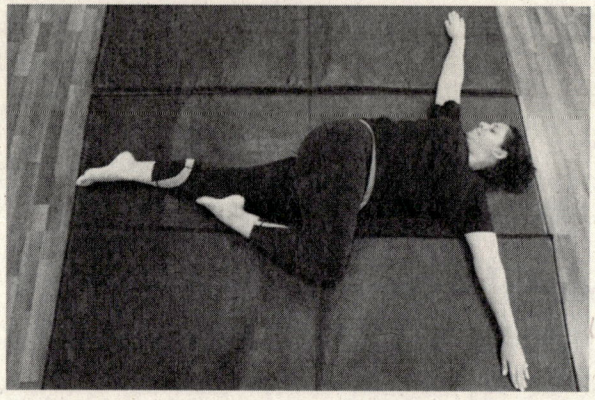

Lie in the supine position, with both legs together and palms resting on the floor. Then spread your arms shoulder level apart and bend your right knee, putting the right foot on the left thigh. With the right knee facing upwards, slowly bring your right knee towards the left side while twisting your back towards the right side and neck to the right as well. Hold for some time, breathing normally, and come back to the original position. Repeat the same on the other side.

Kati Chakrasana Crocodile Series 2

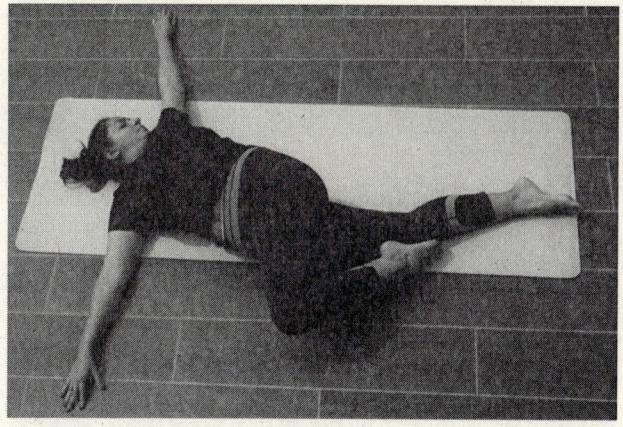

Lie in the supine position, with both legs together and palms resting on the floor. Spread the arms apart in the same distance as between the shoulders, with palms resting on the floor. Now bend your right knee, placing the right foot on the left knee with the right knee facing upwards. Slowly bring your right knee towards the left side while twisting your back towards the right side and neck to the opposite side. Hold the position, breathing normally. Come back to the starting position and repeat the process with the other side.

Kati Chakrasana Crocodile Series 3

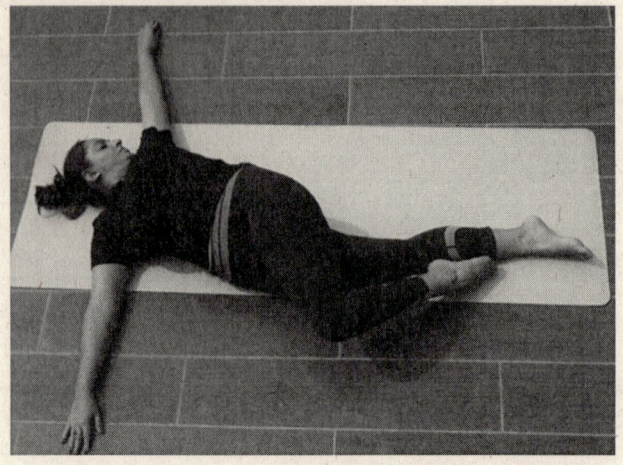

Lie in the supine position, with both legs together and palms resting on the floor. Spread the arms apart in the same distance as between the shoulders, with palms resting on the floor. Bend your right knee, placing the right foot on the left shin (below the knee) and the right knee facing upwards. Slowly bring your right knee towards the left side while twisting your back towards the right side and neck to the opposite side. Hold this position for some time, breathing normally. Come back to the starting position slowly and repeat the process on the other side.

Kati Chakrasana Crocodile Series 4

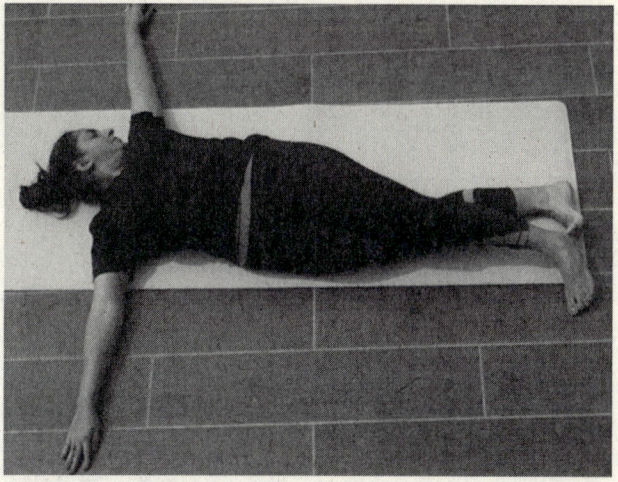

Lie in the supine position, with both legs together and palms resting on the floor. Spread the arms apart in the same distance as between the shoulders, with palms resting on the floor. Now raise the right leg and put the right heel in between the big and the small toe of the left leg while twisting your back towards the left side. Try to touch the floor with the right toe towards the left side, making the neck turn to the opposite side. Hold this position, breathing normally. Come back to the starting position and repeat the same process on the other side.

Kati Chakrasana Crocodile Series 5

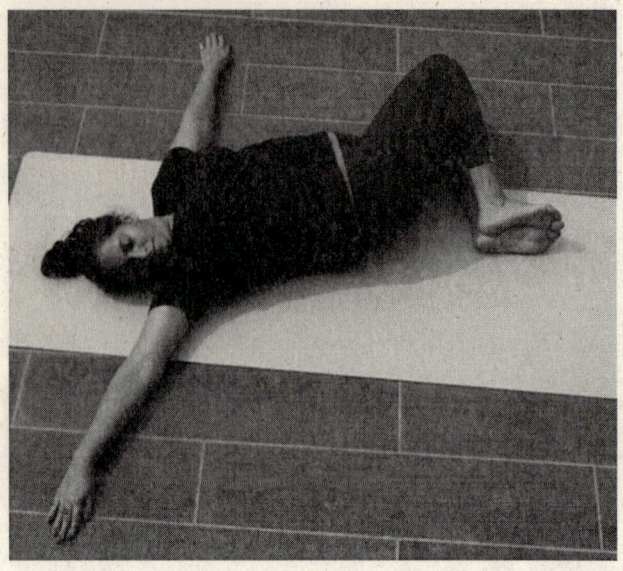

Lie in the supine position, with both legs together and palms resting on the floor. Spread the arms apart in the same distance as between the shoulders, with palms resting on the floor. Now bend both the knees together, then slowly bring the knees towards the left side while twisting the back and turning the neck to the right side. Hold it in this position, breathing normally. Slowly come back to the starting position and repeat the same on the other side.

Kati Chakrasana Crocodile Series 6

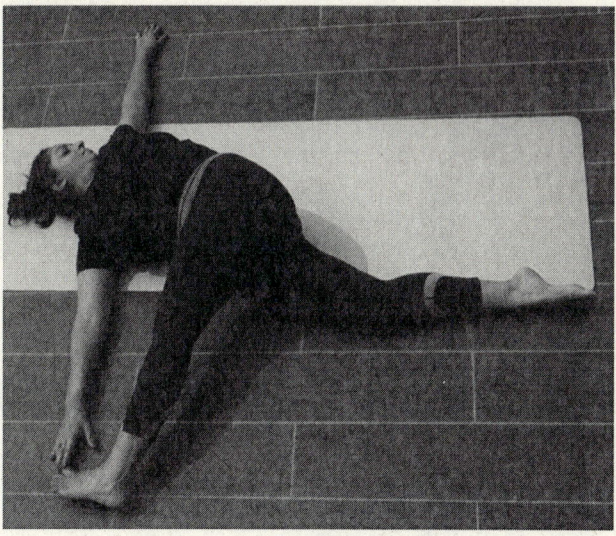

Lie in the supine position, with both legs together and palms resting on the floor. Spread the arms apart in the same distance as between the shoulders, with palms resting on the floor. Now raise the right leg at an angle of 90 degrees from the floor and slowly bring the right foot towards the left side on the floor without bending the right knee but twisting the back and turning the neck to the right side. Hold this position, breathing normally, then come back to the starting position. Repeat process with the other side.

Yog Nidra

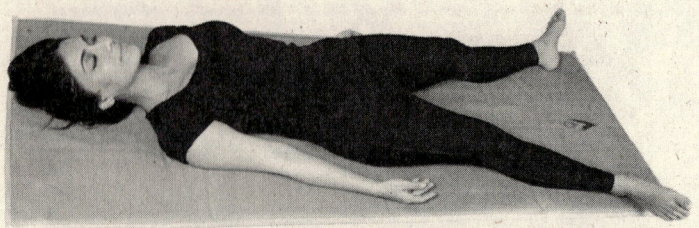

Take the Shavasana position. Now imagine a white ball of light on your crown chakra, that is above your head. The bright ball of light is now entering your body, part by part, moving down to your face, your forehead, nose, lips and chin that are covered with the white light. Moving down the neck, shoulders, arms, palms and fingers; your hands are now covered by the white light. Relax and move the light to your chest, slowly moving to the abdomen and the pelvic region, covering it all with the white light. Move the light to your thighs, calves, ankles, to your feet and your toes. Your entire body is now covered with the white light. Hold it there and relax for a minute, absorbing the light everywhere. Absorb the positive white light and connect with your baby inside you. Then slowly, move the light back in the reverse direction, from the toes, soles of your feet, ankles, calves, thighs, pelvis, abdomen, chest, fingers, arms to your shoulders, neck, chin, nose, ears, and forehead to the crown of your head. The white light has strengthened your protection and with gratitude you can release the white light. Slowly open your eyes and sit up, using your right side.

Sukhasana

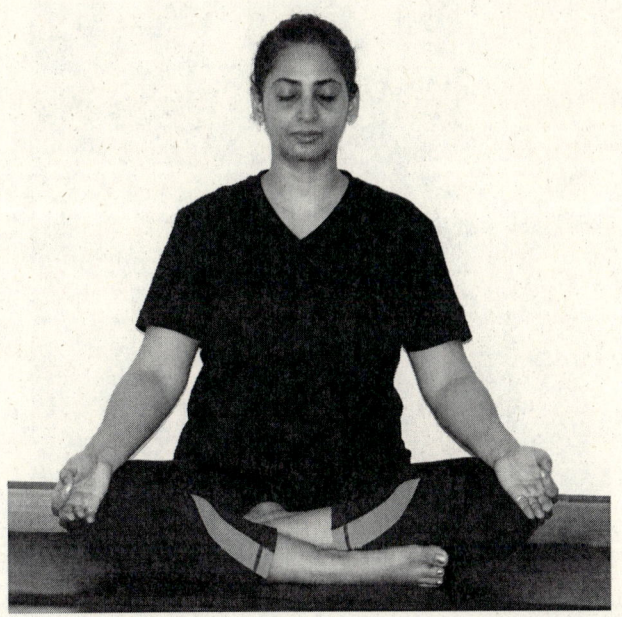

Sit straight with your legs outstretched, keeping the feet together. Cross your shins and slip each foot under the opposite knee while folding the legs towards your body. Keep your back straight. Place your hands on your knees or keep your fingers in a meditative posture (as shown). Breathe normally. Chant Om 10 times in this posture and relax.

Benefits: This helps to relieve tensions from all body parts while relaxing and focusing on each breath. It helps get rid of mood swings and irritability.

Cross-legged Chest Lift

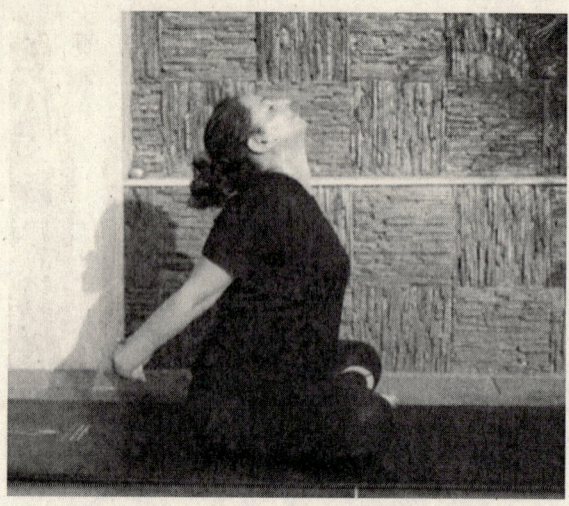

Sit comfortably on the floor and cross your legs. Reach back with both your hands and support yourself on your fingertips, keeping your fingers slightly bent. Inhale and press down gently on your hands to lift up your chest. Look up diagonally and breathe for 4 breath cycles; then relax. Repeat 2 more times.

Benefits: Improves digestion, relieves any strain on the spine caused by prolonged sitting.

Brahma Mudra (see p. 59)

Deep Breathing (see p. 58)

Anulom Vilom (see p. 60)

Om Chanting

Myths

1. Morning sickness may mean reduced nutrition.
2. Eating hot and spicy food causes an abortion.
3. Exercise will harm the baby.
4. Pregnant mothers crave ice cream and pickles.
5. Pregnant mothers should eat for two.

Truth

1. Most common symptoms of pregnancy in the first trimester happen due to hormonal changes.
2. In excess, hot, spicy food may cause heartburn but in moderation, it's safe.
3. After consulting your doctor and having a professional coach you, exercise can actually prepare you for the coming months.
4. Cravings are normal due to the hormonal changes but particular cravings are not universal in nature.
5. It is important to eat a balanced diet, as prescribed by your doctor, and not just increase the quantity of food.

Must Eat

At this point of time, new mothers like to know what is healthy and good for the baby, instead of a diet plan. What to avoid during this period and what will be beneficial can always be advised by your doctor, depending on individual cases. Here are a few items which I followed through during my first trimester:

1. Protein: Spinach, broccoli, eggs, lean meat (chicken), nuts (differ from dry fruits), paneer, cheese
2. Vitamin D: Walnuts, dal (lentils), pomegranates, citrus fruits like oranges, limes
3. Iron: Fish (salmon and cod), beans, yoghurt, black grapes and dates
4. Calcium: Milk, dairy products, sesame seeds, dry fruits (figs)
5. Fibre: Banana, oats, pears, figs, coconut, black beans, peas
6. Folic acid: Almonds, dark green vegetables (okra), bananas

What I avoided during this trimester:

1. Shellfish (crabs/prawns/oysters)
2. Raw papaya/ripe papaya
3. Raw meats
4. Processed food
5. Caffeine
6. King mackerel
7. All refrigerated meats
8. Salads kept on a shelf for long
9. Canned juices
10. Aerated drinks

3

Second Trimester

This is the time you say goodbye to the morning sickness you suffered from in the first trimester as all of it will gradually subside during this time. Things start to get a lot easier and you enjoy this time the most. There's nothing more joyous in this entire universe than seeing your baby bump and feeling your baby move for the first time. Weeks 13 to 28 of the pregnancy is called the second trimester.

For me, it was more of an emotional time where I was full of raging emotions and anything would make me cry at a drop of a hat. I clearly remember that I cried like a baby a few times during this period. I remember realizing the fact that my whole world was about to change and my head was filled with happy thoughts of what I imagined my future was going to be. My husband, Manish, was so ecstatic during my entire pregnancy that I knew that my baby had everything—a loving home, a caring family and proud doting parents; what more could anyone ask for. It is normal for a woman to have happy thoughts and be scared during her pregnancy. First-time mothers go through the phase where everything about their body is different and the mood swings take a toll. I would watch a movie and sob over any love story. Little things like that would tick me off.

Those mothers-to-be who haven't had the chance to enjoy their pregnancy till now will start feeling more energetic about getting things done. At 20 weeks, your doctor does the second ultrasound scan and your blood tests to see if everything looks fine—if your baby is growing and developing as per the required rate or if there is anything to be concerned about.

During the second trimester, there are some symptoms like heart burn and constipation that continue through the next few months and can get worrisome, but as I have always mentioned, please inform your doctor when it gets too bad for you to manage.

Symptoms in the Second Trimester

1. Leg cramps.
2. Swollen feet and ankles.
3. Mouth issues like sensitive gums.
4. Shortness of breath: Due to your growing uterus pushing against the lungs, leaving less space for the flow of air in and out.
5. Stretch marks: On your growing tummy you might notice little white marks. Don't worry as there are many remedies as well as over-the-counter creams, which your doctor will prescribe.

6. Increase in sexual urge: This happens because your body is producing an excessive amount of oestrogen during this time. Usually the mother produces twice the amount of oestrogen during pregnancy, of what she produces in a normal year.

The second trimester is when you start showing and keep growing and growing and growing. I think about the bump as an inflating balloon. This is the time I enjoyed being pampered and being spoilt by my mother. I enjoyed the attention people gave me and all the compliments I received. This was a great instant boost to my mood. The energetic you will want to start preparations for the baby. Errands like shopping for your changing body and for the baby become necessary. When I stepped into my second trimester, the first thing that came to my mind was: Gosh! I am not going to fit into my clothes any more. I remember my husband being supportive of my shopping for the first time in my life. At this time you would need to invest in comfortable maternity clothes, pregnancy panties and bras as well as comfortable footwear.

By this time, your baby is now the size of a pear. This second phase begins at 13 weeks and ends at 28 weeks. You will feel the baby's movements and kicks during this trimester. The baby has developed its coordination skills where it can easily move, giving you sudden jerks and kicks. At this point, almost all mothers say that their child is going to become a football player, because of all the sudden kicks and movements. From here on, the baby starts putting on weight as it grows and hence, so does the mother. The baby grows twice the earlier size during this trimester.

Changes in the Baby

By week 17, the baby's heart is developed and has started to beat independently in coordination with the brain. He/she will be able to move his/her eyelids. The baby's eyes, nose, fingers and ears become more developed, making it easier to hear, smell, see and feel as the eyes are just beginning to open.

The baby has now developed its own digestive system and is able to swallow and even suck his/her thumb. This is a natural behaviour where Mother Nature takes it onto herself to prepare the little one to adapt to the outside world once it's born. The baby also starts growing tiny strands of hair, nails, eyebrows and eyelashes. Even the body will grow a thin coat of hair to help protect the baby and keep her/him warm.

This time every craving you have is actually because of what the baby can taste. As our elders used to say, if you have a liking for a specific food, your baby can grow up to like that food. Never fight your cravings because it's your baby's requirement, more than yours. The baby can actually taste the food that you eat through the amniotic fluid. The cravings didn't really hit me till my cook went on leave in the month of May in 2011. My friend Nazneen and her two daughters came to live with me during that period. She is an excellent cook and her mutton biryani is to die for.

So, even though usually I avoided mutton, I asked her to prepare some the first week she was with me. By the end of her stay, I realized that I had requested her to make that mutton biryani every week.

Changes a Mother Experiences

As I mentioned earlier, many symptoms subside during this time but a few new ones crop up like heartburn, due to the rising levels of hormones related to pregnancy.

Swelling: Young mothers start experiencing this in the second trimester, usually at 22 weeks and it continues till delivery.

What you can do: I advise all mothers to keep their legs elevated at any given chance. Even while sleeping, try and sleep on your side. Wear comfortable footwear when walking and forget about all those fancy shoes and strappy sandals because your feet are really going to swell up! Avoid too much salt and pickles, sour foods, papads and salted chips as this would aggravate the situation.

Dental issues: Many women suffer from dental issues like swollen gums and bleeding gums, which are absolutely normal, but it is very important to inform your doctor if it's too problematic.

What you can do: As dental issues are common in pregnant women, if the intake of calcium is too little, the body starts absorbing what is available, resulting in weak bones. Avoid drinking acidic drinks, from sodas (diet or regular) to Gatorade or sports drinks, which will dissolve the hard surface of the tooth. Gastric reflux and vomiting will also erode the enamel and weaken the teeth so chew sugar-free xylitol gum before you brush your teeth. That way, you don't end up brushing the acid harder into the tooth, causing more wear.

Giddiness: You might feel very lightheaded and dizzy sometimes. It may be due to low blood pressure.

What you can do: Drinking loads of water and having a snack at regular intervals helps. Make sure your meals are not too far apart and that you aren't keeping yourself hungry for long hours. A pregnant woman must eat something every two hours and should stay well-hydrated at all times.

Cramps: Some women start to face this from the 3rd month, right up until the last. The leg cramps happen due to the pregnancy hormones along with the added weight, and deficiency in magnesium and calcium.

What you can do: The only remedy for this is a good healthy diet. Don't cut down on fatty foods or carbs. A healthy diet is very important so follow what is suggested by your doctor.

Lower tummy aches: This happens due to not wearing supportive protection for your growing tummy. It is basically the ligaments that ache when they are not supported well.

What you can do: Wear clothing with comfortable stretchable waistbands. This is available at all undergarment stores and also online. Always make sure you are sitting in a comfortable position at all times. Do not strain your back or add extra pressure as this could aggravate the situation.

Varicose veins/spider veins, haemorrhoids: This problem is a common issue some women face during pregnancy. It usually happens anywhere from the waist down like on your thighs, feet ankles, vulva, rectum; when the nerves around your rectum swell-up, it is known as haemorrhoids. This is a result of your body providing excess amount of blood for you and your baby which sometimes results in putting excess pressure on your blood vessels, especially in the lower body area due to the constant pressure from your body on your legs. This happens again because of the pregnancy hormone called progesterone which relaxes the vein vessels, making circulation through the body back to the heart slow down, resulting in excess pressure in these areas. They ache or itch sometimes but usually shrink or completely go away after delivery in most cases.

What you can do: Ointments and medications are given for them to subside. In most cases it is hereditary and can be passed on so be sure that if your mother had it then you might just get them as well. Also, for those who experienced it in their first pregnancy, the situation can worsen as these veins can cause clots if not treated by your doctor. It is very important to increase the circulation in these areas. I advise all mothers to wear comfortable footwear and not to sit cross-legged for a long time. Whenever possible, relax your feet and keep them well-elevated. Use a stool in office and pillows under your legs when in bed. Another important thing to keep in mind is to sleep on the left side as much as possible as it reduces the pressure on your main blood vessels and aids in good circulation. For those who are overweight, I would recommend keeping a check on your weight and maintaining a healthy balanced diet. Weight puts a whole lot of strain on your growing body. For those who feel that their varicose veins haven't improved or gone after birth, seek medical help. With new technology and advances in science and medicine, there are many solutions available, so do not worry.

Sex during Pregnancy

One of the most queried issues, sex is always a dicey topic during pregnancy. My doctor had informed me that I was going to experience many different changes and my mood swings will get the best of me. For many women, first accepting that their body is changing is a big deal. It takes time for a woman to get over it and for her to be more confident with her partner. There are days when your partner is in the mood but you feel sick and tired. During this time, it is important to have a good communication system. You need to speak up and make your partner understand how you feel.

Prenatal education is easily available online and you could also speak to your doctor who could help you out. This doesn't mean you cannot have sex at all during pregnancy. Most partners are scared to have penetrative intercourse because they feel they are hurting the baby or the mother, but doctors will assure you that nothing is wrong with it and sometimes the baby may even enjoy the rocking movements. The doctor will inform you about the best and most comfortable postures.

Sex is known to reduce blood pressure, which is beneficial for the mother and child. After a good lovemaking session, get a good night's sleep, as this helps burn calories and relaxes the mother and the baby.

Dealing with Weight Gain

Many women tend to get conscious about the sudden weight gain as it is common to put on anywhere from 2 to 5 kilograms during this time. Some feel that, since the frequency of meals has increased, the weight will also increase rapidly. There is no reason to worry as the quantity you eat is also broken down so you are basically eating for yourself and your baby.

Let us learn how Sunaina faced her pregnancy weight gain. Sunaina was a happily married 26-year-old, working at an IT company in the human resources department. She learnt that she was pregnant after some of the symptoms, mentioned in the earlier chapters, showed up. She and her husband were delighted and they started planning for the coming months. They invited her parents to come over and stay with them for some time. Her parents were very happy and did everything they could to make this period comfortable for the couple. Sunaina soon started gaining weight as her food intake increased and her job afforded her almost no time for exercise. Her doctor advised her to take some time off and concentrate on her diet so that she did not develop any symptoms which come with above normal weight gain during pregnancy. She followed the doctor's instructions. After a healthy delivery, Sunaina decided to work hard to get back to her fitness level. It took her a while, with yoga and general exercise along with taking care of the baby, before she reached her weight goal. Three years later, when she was pregnant with her second child, she was careful about her diet and exercise regime, and did not indulge her cravings too much so that she could keep her weight at a healthy level for herself and the baby.

Exercise plays an important role in the second trimester in pregnancy and will help you manage your extra kilos. It helps in knocking them off easily later. I always say that walking and a good amount of swimming wouldn't hurt you, although overexertion is never recommended. Exercise is always advised only once your doctor feels you are ready for it. Please speak to your doctor before starting any kind of exercise, keeping in mind that some sports are not advised.

Dos and Don'ts

1. Drink plenty of water during your pregnancy as this flushes out toxins stored in the body, making it easy on the bowel system.

2. Avoid caffeine during pregnancy.
3. Avoid junk food.
4. Do not overeat.
5. Do not overdo your exercise routine.
6. Take vitamins and other medications as prescribed by your doctor on time.
7. Do not stand for long hours.
8. Avoid strenuous work.
9. Avoid overcrowded spaces.
10. Try and go for walks in the morning for a breath of fresh air for 20 minutes at least, at a slow pace.
11. Do not drink alcohol or smoke.
12. Avoid being in the same room as people who are smoking.
13. Avoid uncooked sea food like sushi.

Pregnancy Week by Week

Week 13: At this point, your baby is the size of a peach and is about 3 inches long. Your baby's head has now grown in proportion to its body. At 13 weeks your baby can swallow and urinate.

Week 14: Your baby is the size of a lemon. At this stage, your baby can use his/her facial muscles and on a 3D ultrasound you can catch those cute smiles and frowns, and if you're lucky, you can even see the baby sucking his/her finger.

Week 15: The baby has reached the shape of an apple, and is about 4 inches long. The eyes are still shut, though he/she can sense light and if you flash a torchlight, it might just get really excited and start moving away.

Week 16: Your baby resembles an avocado at this point and is about 5 inches long. The neck is starting to hold up in position at this point as the spine muscles are getting stronger.

Week 17: The baby is now about 140 gm and is the size of a pear. His/her hearing is developing at this stage and the body is getting much stronger compared to its rubbery structure initially.

Week 18: Your baby is now the size of a capsicum weighing about 190 gm. He/she can flex arms and legs by this time, so watch out for sudden movements which are going to get more regular.

Week 19: At 19 weeks your baby is the size of a mango, weighing about 240 gm. The baby starts developing tiny strands of hair on the head. At this point, he/she can hear your voice and get excited. The sensory organs are much more developed at this point which makes it a crazy time for the baby.

Week 20: Your baby is the size of a coconut and weighs 300 gm. The development at this stage is of the sex of the baby. If it's a girl, her vaginal canal is forming whereas if it is a boy it would take time as his genitals are still descending and are still in the abdomen. It'll be a while before its scrotum grows.

Week 21: At 21 weeks your baby is the size of a papaya and weighs 365 gm. He/she has developed taste buds, which means he/she is swallowing amniotic fluids from your tummy. The fluid is built up of nutrients based on the food you eat, therefore what you eat at this point is tasted by the baby. If you want your baby to have a healthy eating habit once he/she is out of your belly, you need to introduce loads of fresh food like fruits and vegetables. Your baby is now growing tiny eyebrows.

Week 22: The baby is the size of a zucchini and weighs around 430 gm. At this point, your baby's movements are much more regular and most of them may feel like sudden jerks when he/she kicks. Babies form a daily living pattern, playing around for some time or taking a nap. You could try and sneak in a nap during that time too.

Week 23: Your baby is just about 30 cm long and is the size of a big mango. The weight would approximately be 500 gm. His/her hearing sense is very distinct at this point, hence, he/she will be able to hear sounds of the outside world which makes it easier for the baby to cope once it is born.

Week 24: He/she is now growing at a rapid speed and is now the size of an ear of corn, weighing 600 gm. At this point, your baby has eyebrows, eyelashes and hair but the pigmentation isn't there at the moment.

Week 25: Your baby is the size of a brinjal and weighs around 660 gm. The lungs have developed and the baby would be able to practise breathing at this time. He/she would be practising with inhaling amniotic fluid but that's all right. He/she could get excited by certain sounds like music or even other people's voices.

Week 26: Your baby is the size of a long cucumber and weighs 760 gm now. Your baby has now grown finger nails which will be visible and long when they're born. At this time, your baby might feel cramped but don't worry, the uterus will grow to accommodate your little one. You will notice the toss and turn little less and slower movements, which would be visible through your tight-fitting clothes.

Week 27: The baby is now the size of a cauliflower and weighs 875 gm. At this point, his/her sense of taste is extremely distinct, which means anything sour or spicy would send the baby into a bout of hiccups, but that's all right and isn't an immediate response. It usually takes place more than 90 minutes after you have eaten.

Yoga for the Second Trimester

Before beginning the workout, prepare in the following manner:

The place: Choose a place which has fresh air and is well circulated, preferably a garden, a terrace, or a workout place in your house. If the place is indoors, try gentle lighting in the room.

The requirements: A yoga mat, a bottle of water, a hand or face towel. You can play some slow music in the background if you like.

To start: Spread the mat on the floor and sit in a comfortable position. Take five to ten long breaths to relax yourself. Stretch your hands and legs to loosen the muscles. Perform the warm-up exercises mentioned in Chapter 1 (p. 14), without putting any undue stress on your body.

Side Leg Kick

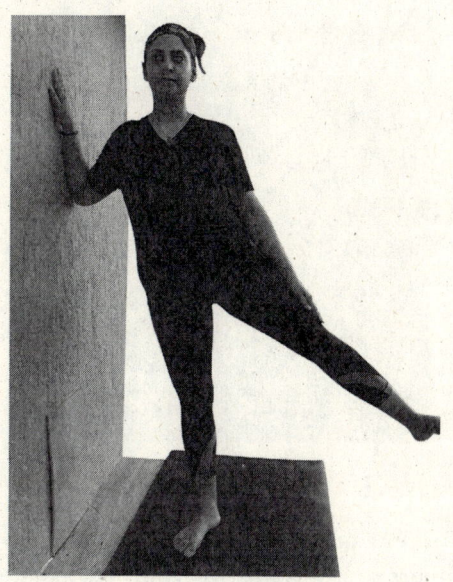

Stand beside a wall with one shoulder at a hand-distance gap from the wall. Take the support of the wall with your left hand. Lift your right leg sideways as much as you can and slowly bring it down; then repeat this, taking your leg up again and bringing it down slowly. Breathe normally and repeat this 10 times. Do this with the other leg. Come back to the start and relax.

Benefits: This helps relieve oedema (fluid retention) and cramping which is quite common in the last months.

Forward Leg Kick

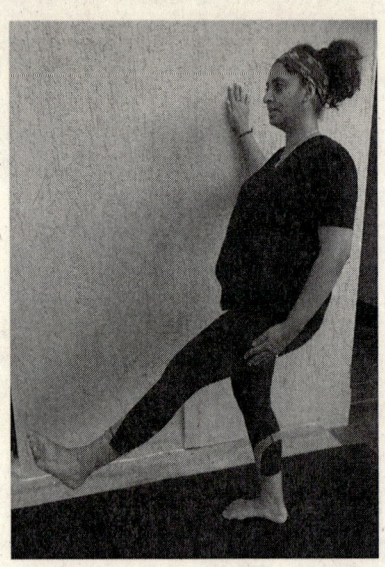

Stand beside a wall with shoulders at a hand-distance gap. Take the support of the wall with your left hand. Lift your right leg forward as much as you can and slowly bring it down. Now repeat this, taking your leg up again and bringing it down slowly while breathing normally. Repeat this 10 times, breathing normally. Do this with the other leg. Come back to the start and relax.

Benefits: This helps relieve oedema (fluid retention) and cramping which can be quite common in the last months.

Backward Leg Kick

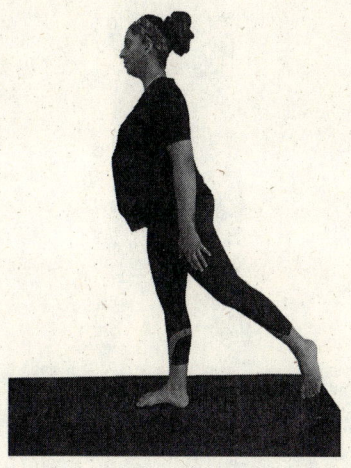

Stand beside a wall with shoulders at a hand-distance gap. Take the support of the wall with your left hand. Lift your right leg backwards as much as you can and slowly bring it down; repeat this, taking your leg up again and bringing it down slowly while breathing normally. Repeat this 10 times, breathing normally. Do this with the other leg. Come back to the start and relax.

Benefits: This helps relieve oedema (fluid retention) and cramping which can be quite common in the last months.

Kati Chakrasana (Waist-rotating Pose)

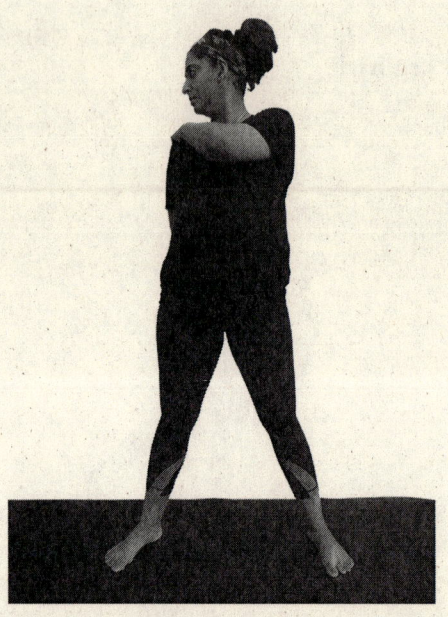

Stand with your feet about half a metre apart and your arms by your side. Inhale while raising the arms to shoulder level. Exhale and twist body to left. Bring your right hand to the left shoulder and wrap the left arm around the back. Look over the left shoulder. Hold your breath for 2 seconds, inhale and return to the starting position. Keep your feet firmly on the ground while twisting. Repeat on the other side. Twist smoothly without any jerks. Do about 5–10 rounds.

Benefits: Tones the waist, back and hips. Induces a feeling of lightness and relieves physical and mental tension.

Saral Santolasana

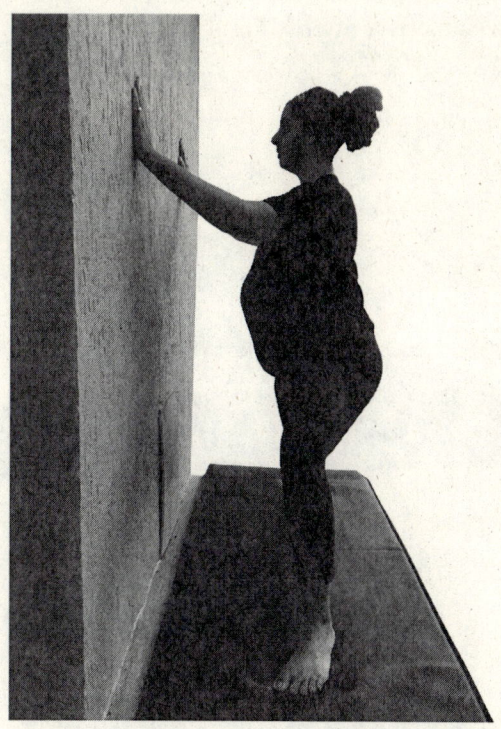

Stand while facing the wall with your feet apart and at an arms-distance from the wall. Put your palms on the wall and try to push the wall with your hands, bending at the elbow, and make the contraction on your hand do a push-up against the wall 15-20 times, breathing normally.

Benefits: Helps develop physical and mental balance and strengthens the upper body. The entire spine and back are stretched and loosened, helping to clear congestion of the spinal nerves.

Marjari Asana (Cat Stretch Pose)

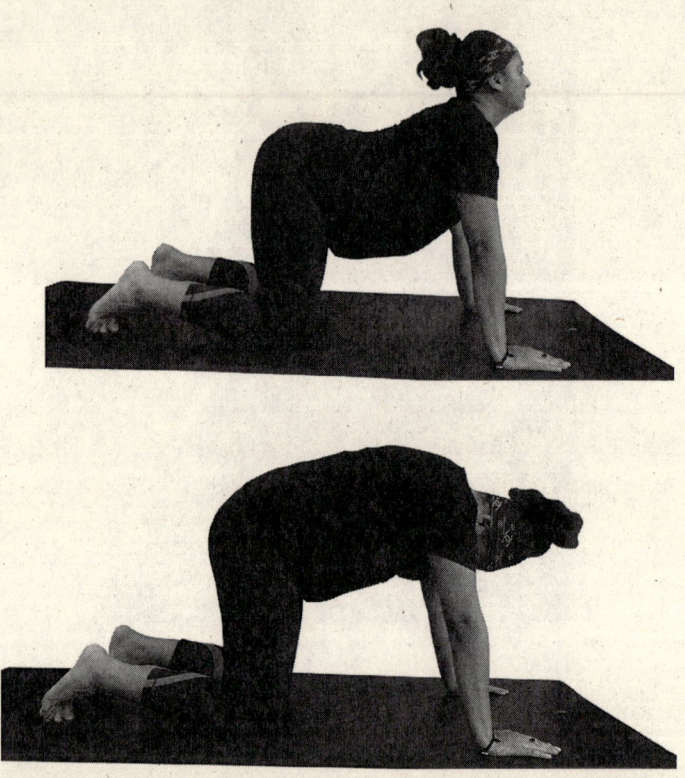

Sit with your buttocks on your heels (Vajrasana). Raise your buttocks and stand on your knees. Lean forward and place your hands flat on the floor. This is the starting position. Inhale while raising your head. Exhale while lowering your head and stretching the spine upwards. At the end of the exhalation, pull in the buttocks. Your head will now be between the arms, facing the thighs. This is one round. It may be performed 5–10 times. Be careful not to strain yourself.

Benefits: This asana improves the flexibility of the neck, shoulders and spine. It also tones the female reproductive system.

Ardha Titali Asana (Half Butterfly Pose)

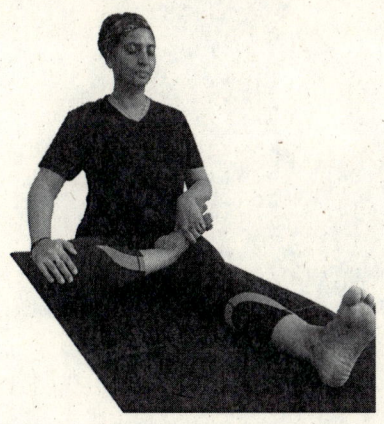

Stretch your legs in front of you as you sit. Bend the right leg by placing the right foot as far up on the left as possible. Keep your right hand on top of the bent right knee. Use your left hand to hold the toes of the right foot. Gently move the right knee up towards the chest while breathing in. While breathing out, gently push the knee down and try to touch the floor. The trunk should not move. Movement of the leg should be achieved by the exertion of the right arm. Repeat with the left leg. Slowly practise about 10 up and down movements with each leg. Do not strain.

Benefits: To make your hip and knee joints a bit more flexible, this is an excellent exercise.

Poorna Titali Asana (Full Butterfly Pose)

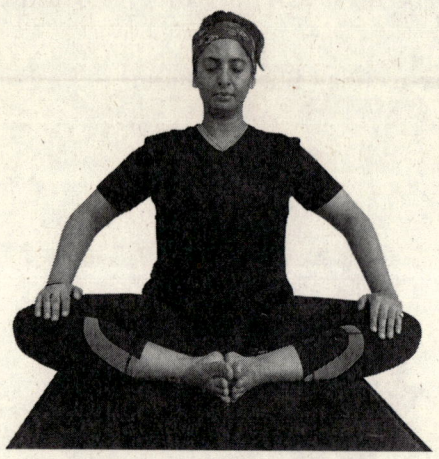

Sit against a wall with your legs outstretched. Bend the knees and bring the soles of the feet together, keeping the heels as close to the body as possible. Fully relax the inner thighs. Rest your palms on your knees while keeping the shoulders straight and elbows bent. Do not use any force. Repeat up to 20–30 times. Straighten the legs and relax.

Benefits: Tension from the inner thigh muscles is relieved. Helps reduce tiredness in the legs.

Matsya Kridasana (Flapping Fish Pose)

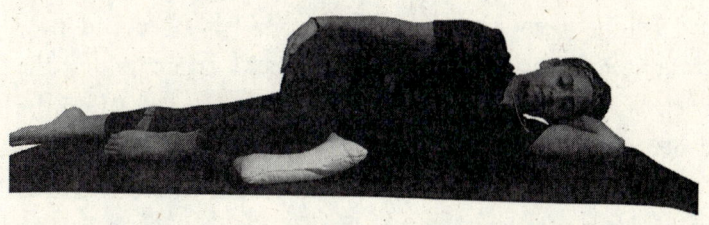

Lie on your side (you could use a pillow for comfort) with your left hand under your head or whichever way is comfortable for you. Bend the right leg sideways and bring the right knee close to the body. The left leg should remain straight. Relax in the final pose, and after some time, change sides. The bent knee and head may be supported on a pillow for further comfort.

Benefits: Stimulates digestion and removes constipation. It relaxes nerves of the legs.

Lying Hamstring Stretch

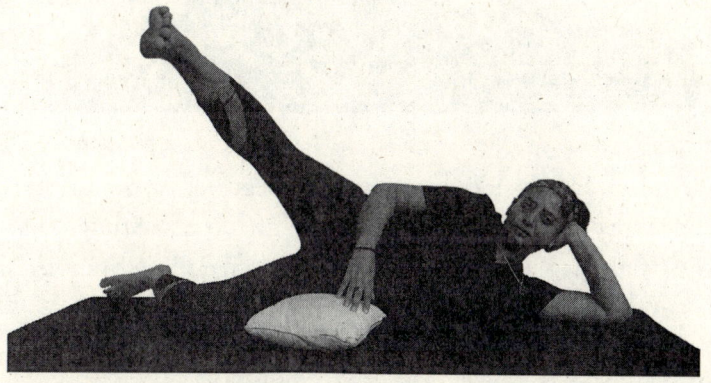

Lie on your left side with a pillow under your stomach for your comfort. Keeping your head up or lying on the bed according to your comfort, fold your left knee and now straighten your left knee forward. Feel a stretch along the back of your leg and hold for 4 breath cycles. Repeat on the other side.

Benefits: Relaxes the hamstring, groin muscles and abdominal muscles, making them more flexible and more comfortable for the baby.

Lying Inner Thigh Stretch

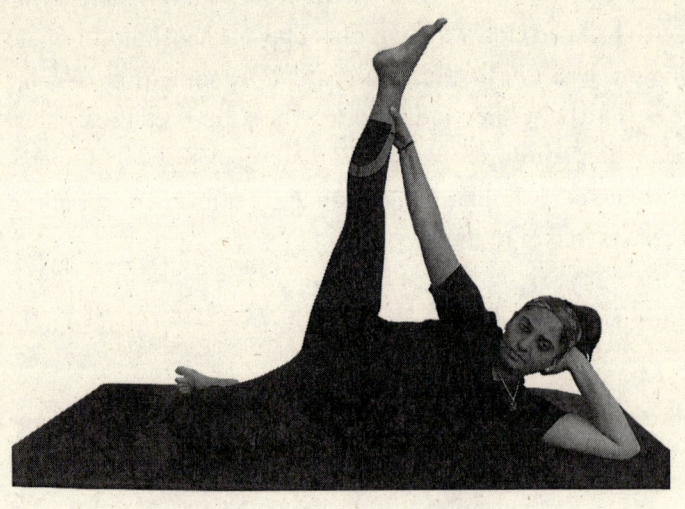

Lie on your left side, keeping your head up or lie on the bed. Now slightly bend both legs at the knees. Straighten your right leg and grasp your knee and pulling your leg towards you as much as you can, feel a stretch inside your thighs. Now hold for 3 breath cycles; repeat on the other side.

Benefits: Focuses on relieving tension around the cervix and birth canal.

Lying Quad Stretch

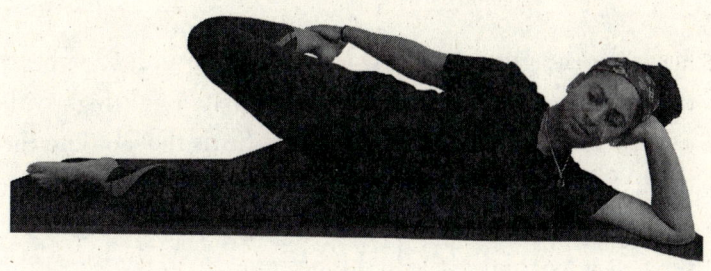

Lie on your left side, keeping your head up or lie on the bed. Slightly bend your left leg. Tuck your pelvis under as you reach back to grasp your right ankle or shin and gently pull towards your buttock. Feel a comfortable stretch in the front of your right thigh. Hold for 3 breath cycles. Repeat on the other side.

Benefits: Makes the legs more flexible and focuses on opening up the pelvis to make labour easier and quicker.

Ardha Padmasana

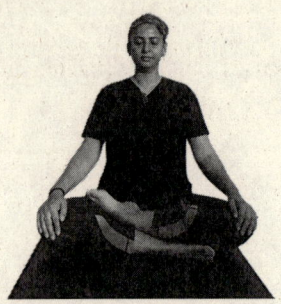

Sit on a mat against a wall with your legs forward. Now bend the left knee and bring the left ankle to the right thigh with the sole of the left foot facing upwards. Settle the foot into the thigh. Bend the right knee and cross the right ankle under the left knee/shin in a comfortable, cross-legged position. Sit in the pose for some time. Now, in this posture, do Ashwin Mudra.

Ashwin Mudra

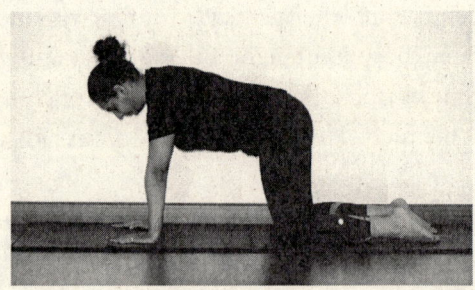

In cat pose, while inhaling, expand your anus muscles outwards and while exhaling, contract your anus muscles inwards. Repeat this 10–15 times. Relax your body and breathe normally.

Benefits: It helps strengthen weak pelvic muscles and ease constipation.

Myths

1. Depending on how you carry your baby, you can determine the sex of the baby.
2. If you raise your hands above your head, the baby will get the cord wrapped around its neck.
3. If you have a lot of heartburn during pregnancy, the baby will be born with a lot of hair.
4. Stormy weather or the full moon can initiate labour.

Truth

1. How you carry your baby is affected by the time of the year when you are pregnant, your height and weight. The sex of the baby has nothing to do with it.
2. That's not at all true. No form of exercise contributes to the cord getting wrapped around any part of the baby.
3. This is not necessary. You should let your doctor know if you suffer from heartburn during pregnancy.
4. It's not a scientific fact.

Must Eat

Those who cannot do without tea should not have more than 1½ cups a day. As a treat you can have some dark chocolate as it contains magnesium, potassium, iron and calcium. Here are a few items which I increased during my second trimester:

1. Calcium: Ragi, milk and dairy products, and dry fruits
2. Vitamin D: Cereals, orange juice, egg yolks, salmon (rawas) and mackerel (surmai)
3. Magnesium: It is very important as it helps prevent premature contractions in the uterus. Increase intake of green and leafy vegetables: spinach, okra (bhindi), legumes (dals), grains, oats, brown rice, nuts (almonds, peanuts, hazelnuts), bananas
4. Seeds: Sunflower and pumpkin
5. Fibre : Soya bean, broccoli, oats, banana
6. Omega 3 foods: Flax seeds (reduces bloating) and walnuts

What I avoided during this trimester:

1. Papaya and pineapple
2. Tea/coffee
3. Tulsi leaves
4. Arbi, as it causes bloating.
5. Heat-producing foods like methi, til, dates, ajwain, besan.

4

Third Trimester

This is the beginning of the seventh month where you feel like your growing belly can't get any bigger. I assure you that it is, in fact, going to get bigger! Having finally reached the 28th-week mark, an expecting mother has entered into the 3rd trimester. This is when you can make the most of your precious nap times because in just a few weeks you will need to start preparing for the arrival of your baby. There are many changes that you will still go through and there are many things people haven't told you about giving birth, but don't be alarmed. It's all worth it. Once you see and hold your little baby, you forget every pain, ache and unpleasant memory of nausea you went through. All the waddling to the loo in the middle of the night drove me crazy but it's totally worth it and I wouldn't mind doing it again.

I remember being so confused when I entered my 3rd trimester because what I read in pregnancy books and what

I read online were different theories. Some said that the 26th week, some say the 27th and some, the 28th week was the beginning of the third trimester. The best is to consult your doctor and stick to what your doctor says. I and my husband tried spending most of our time together during this period as we knew our lives would become busy once the baby came, and I didn't want to neglect my husband. He understood this, but during those weeks, these silly thoughts would give me anxiety. Would we be good parents? Would we be able to look after every need of the baby? There are many things that keep coming to mind, especially for those mothers who suffer from pregnancy insomnia.

Women who suffer from pregnancy insomnia are more prone to being exhausted, and suffer from aches, pain and extreme anxiety because even though their body is tired, they are unable to have a good night's sleep. In the third trimester, the pressure on the mother's lungs increases which makes her feel exhausted but not comfortable enough to sleep. I remember many sleepless, uncomfortable nights when finding a comfortable position to sleep became very difficult along with the almost constant need to pee due to the pressure on my bladder. You need to contact your doctor for advice on how to take care of yourself and get adequate rest.

Do not take over-the-counter medications without the doctor's advice. It is very important to keep this in mind as whatever you do can affect the baby in some way or the other. By this time the womb feels as if it is cramped, causing a lot of discomfort for your internal organs and for your baby, which will, in turn, make you more tired and exhausted quicker. For me, my prenatal yoga came in handy. My yoga routine while being pregnant, which I have added at the end of this chapter, made it easier for me by giving me more stamina and reduced swelling on my feet.

You might feel anxious as the day gets closer and you start preparing for the arrival of the baby. Exhaustion is going to get the best of you in the coming months and what you feel you could complete in an hour's time before might take you three hours now. There are many different changes women face in the third trimester that can be extreme. I put on the most weight during my third trimester. I also experienced a lot of swelling and water retention which made me look as if I was carrying twins!

When my neighbour was in her third trimester, she suffered from an extreme case of haemorrhoids, which were so painful that it made it hard for her to pass a normal stool. She even found daily activities like sitting and walking uncomfortable and painful because it used to itch and pain. This happens to women who have had the problem earlier, making it worse. They tend to happen in the second trimester and worsen in the third or start straight away in the third trimester.

This happens due to the hormone progesterone whose levels increase in the body during pregnancy. When this hormone is produced in excess, it relaxes the vein walls, making them inflamed and more prone to swelling. This, in turn, contributes to constipation by making it harder to pass the interstitial tract. This constipation makes you strain, which puts more pressure on the veins, making them swell up. If at any time you suffer from this, please inform your doctor, who will prescribe appropriate medications.

Dos and Don'ts for the Third Trimester

1. Drink at least 2 litres of water a day to avoid constipation.
2. Include foods with fibre like fruits, raw vegetables, beans, whole grains.
3. Sleep on your left side and never on your back. Use a pillow between your legs and one behind you to support your back. This helps circulation without putting a strain on the uterus.
4. Do not take your mobile phone with you into the bathroom as this increases the time you sit in the toilet, putting a strain and pressure on your rectal area.
5. Do Kegel exercises as much as possible as this not only helps pelvic blood flow but also strengthens the muscles in that region.
6. Even though it is uncomfortable to walk, avoid sitting or sleeping for long intervals. It is important for you to keep active during this time as you need to relieve pressure on the rectal area.
7. Try and smoothen the area with warm water and cold water a couple of times a day. This relieves the nerves, giving you relief.

Common Problems

- Heartburn
- Braxton Hicks contractions
- Increased foetal movement
- Swelling
- Visiting the loo more often than usual along with leakage
- Haemorrhoids
- Constipation
- Breast tenderness and secretion of fluid
- Sleeping issues

These are some of the problems a mother experiences during this period, and though they might make you feel scared, do not worry because at this point a mother becomes very cautious and forms a defensive motherly instinct towards her belly. In these coming months, you will find yourself touching your tummy more often than usual and being more protective while enjoying the feel of your baby.

You will notice a significant increase in your weight during this trimester. This is because the baby's organs are formed and it is now time for the baby to put on some of its own weight. This is also accompanied by the water and other fluids in the body like an increase in blood, amniotic fluid, the placenta, not to forget the growing uterus.

OTHER CHANGES A MOTHER CAN EXPECT

Bigger breasts: Your breasts have grown bigger and later on, a yellowish liquid is secreted. Do not be alarmed, this is totally normal. Some women think it is an infection of some sort but this yellowish liquid is the baby's first food, which is packed with nutrients and is what helps to build the baby's immunity.

Breathlessness: There are times where you will notice the feeling of breathlessness. This happens because the space to accommodate a baby is very limited, causing the uterus to push against the lungs that in turn causes shortness of breath. The space where the lungs usually inflate while inhaling is reduced due to the size of your uterus, making it difficult to breathe comfortably, giving you short breaths. Do not be scared. You might feel your baby isn't getting enough oxygen, but the lungs start to accommodate the air inside for longer. You could change or correct your posture whenever you feel like this because it is very important for you to maintain a good posture during pregnancy. For that, I recommend yoga with Pranayam, which consists of proper breathing techniques and will help you right up to labour and contractions.

Trouble sleeping: Most women have problems while sleeping. You are not used to having any obstruction when sleeping before pregnancy and when your belly has grown to this size, it gets difficult to find a comfy spot to fall off to sleep. Unable to toss and turn freely will make you feel extremely frustrated. Those who are used to sleeping on their back need to change their sleeping position because the pressure of the baby in the uterus is pushed on to the chest, making it difficult and uncomfortable as well as resulting in low blood circulation in your body.

The ideal posture is to sleep on your left side so that the baby is able to move around more freely. This posture puts less pressure on the heart and helps in better circulation of blood. To make yourself more comfortable, use a pillow between your legs or behind your back for more support.

Indigestion and heartburn: This is due to the pressure of the uterus on the stomach and intestines causing it to push food back up the oesophagus. This can be minimized and avoided by waiting for at least an hour after eating and then lying down. Eat smaller and more frequent meals throughout the day, while never staying hungry for long intervals. Always leave the house with a small box of dry fruits or a fruit, so that if you are stuck somewhere you can munch on something. Eat home-cooked meals with less oil, spices and minimal deep fried stuff as this aggravates the situation. If you suffer from indigestion or heartburn, try drinking some cold milk or eat a few spoons of yoghurt to soothe your system.

Backache: At this time your back must be killing you. The reason is the weight of your growing belly, which is a strain on your back along with the cramped situation inside, where your baby pushes and kicks against your ribs, creating pressure on your chest. With the growing uterus, the pressure builds and presses the sciatic nerve, resulting in backaches. But that's not the only reason. At this stage, your body is also producing a hormone called 'relaxin' which is used to loosen up your joints to make it easier for your baby's delivery, therefore, putting a whole load of strain on your lower back, hips and your tail bone area.

Abdominal pain: There are two different types of pain where one would need medical attention. One could be because of your growing tummy making the skin and everything inside tight (it could be anything from a sharp pain to a tingly sensation), or gas, indigestion, constipation, or even Braxton Hicks. The other can be serious if accompanied with fever, nausea, vaginal bleeding, vomiting and dizziness. This would need immediate medical help.

Braxton Hicks: Dr John Braxton Hicks in 1872 named the mild contractions a woman has before real labour after his name. These contractions usually happen in the second trimester right up to the third. The feeling the mother-to-be experiences during Braxton Hicks is a strong pull of muscles, a tightening in the uterus for anything between a minute or half and can go on for a little longer. During this time, I suggest you make use of all the prenatal breathing techniques you learnt in your yoga class. There are a few reasons why these are triggered. These can happen when the mother hasn't had enough of water, causing dehydration, or when you control your pee and hold on to your full bladder. Women experience this even after sex.

Frequent loo breaks: You will also notice that the frequency of passing urine has increased. During this time your baby is lying squashed in your pelvic area against your bladder, therefore, making it difficult to accommodate a lot of fluids.

Sometimes due to the pressure, you can have a leak which is common even as you bend, laugh or sneeze. At any given time do not stop or lower your water intake. Always stay hydrated as it is very important to maintain the water level in your body.

Cramps: This is more common in the third trimester where your feet, hands, tummy or legs areas are more prone to cramps. This happens usually in the second trimester right up to the third trimester. They say it's because of too much phosphorus and less calcium in the body. Cramps in the tummy are because of the growing uterus which in turn is stretched because of the support provided by the ligaments and muscles. This cramping is noticeably felt, especially when you are in a bad position or crouching. Other reasons for leg cramps are inadequate circulation and the pressure of the baby, which is taking a toll on your legs. It can even happen in your sleep when your leg is flexed too much. Easing your foot out is recommended if it happens when you are sleeping but once you do that, try standing firm on the floor and lift yourself on your toes. You could also massage the area by putting pressure on the affected area and pulling the pain downwards.

Swelling and bloating: Accompanied by gas, this is a common problem. The reason behind this is the excess water retention in the body which makes you swell up like a balloon. This is also called oedema. You will notice your feet, fingers, legs, ankles swollen. Rings don't fit anymore nor can your feet fit into your slippers at times. The reason for this is because of fluids that tend to gather in parts of your body due to the excess weight and pull of gravity. You will notice that it gets worse during the day and by the end of the night. Swelling in the legs due to weight and low blood circulation could also lead to varicose veins, which are also common during the third trimester.

You can blame the high levels of progesterone which has constantly been slowing down your system and enabling the bloating. It relaxes smooth muscle tissue in your body and in your digestive system. This slows down digestion which inadvertently leads to indigestion, gas, constipation, heartburn, burping and so on.

Tips to Soothe Swelling and Bloating

1. Elevate your legs while sleeping or sitting.
2. Do not sit or stand for long hours. Always take a break from either of the activities as this increases the circulation.
3. Cut down on your salt intake as this worsens the situation.
4. Increase your water intake as this helps to flush out toxins which make the body less likely to retain fluids.
5. Cut down sugar-based drinks.
6. Wear loose clothing.
7. Always sit at the table while eating; this will cut down on bad posture while eating, making food easier to digest.
8. Take a walk whenever possible after eating. This will aid in digestion.

Stretch marks: This is one of the most annoying consequences of pregnancy, which some women might suffer from, while others have the most glowing and clear skin. This happens when the skin is stretched not only around the tummy but on the breast and buttocks also. As long as your body is growing in order to accommodate your growing baby, your skin tightens and gets discoloured. This also happens if your mother or grandmother suffered from it during their pregnancies. For this, you could choose a diet rich in vitamins that increase the elasticity of your skin.

Tips to Avoid Stretch Marks

1. Boil rose petals and olive oil for 20 minutes and strain. This can be kept for a month and is to be used to massage into the affected areas or all over during and after pregnancy.
2. Boil aloe vera and coconut oil together for 30 minutes and stir well. Store and apply 3 times a day for best results. (You could start applying it in the first trimester as this increases the elasticity in the skin.)
3. Almond oil is also good for removing stretch marks.

Pregnancy Week by Week

Week 28: It is the beginning of your third trimester. You should be visiting your doctor every two weeks. This is the time when your breasts may secrete colostrum. It is also the baby fat deposition stage.

Week 29: You are well into the third trimester. This is when some women face the problems of indigestion and varicose veins. Your baby is growing and storing energy fat now and is also forming teeth.

Week 30: Some women face heartburn during this time, and sleep disturbance is a common problem. The baby's thermoregulation begins.

Week 31: It's a phase of expansion where the mother notices a decrease in her will to exercise. The baby might be around 1.8 kg and 38–44 cm long.

Week 32: Some mothers may notice hyperpigmentation on her nipples. It means that the sucking reflex of the baby starts becoming stronger.

Week 33: A strong baby may weigh around 2.25 kg.

Week 34: The mother may suffer from swollen feet, heartburn and backache. It's time now for the parents to understand the delivery process and prepare for it. The child may weigh around 2.5 kg and be around 50 cm long, in some cases.

Week 35: This is when you should start keeping your delivery bag ready. The mother can expect only sideways movements now from the baby. The brain of the baby develops at a great pace at this stage. The mother should include plenty of DHA (docosahexaenoic acid) and Omega3 rich food in her diet.

Week 36: Working mothers, who have not yet availed it, should consider going on maternity leave now. Heartburn, breathlessness, and the general feeling of tiredness will increase. The well-being of the mother and baby should be monitored carefully at this time.

Weeks 37–40: Deliveries usually take place during these weeks.

Exercise during the Third Trimester

Many women feel like it's best to rest during the 3rd trimester because a woman's energy levels aren't as high as they used to be. But I always suggest some kind of activity, if not yoga. Now, most doctors suggest prenatal yoga for mothers because of the vast benefits it has to offer. It not only prepares you for pregnancy but also boosts your mood, raises your energy levels and increases your flexibility. These are just a few benefits but yoga helps you get back in shape and lose those extra kilos while toning your body and tightening your stomach.

Yoga has certain asanas that stretch the body, giving it more flexibility, making it easier during the 9 months. Yoga and meditation are the keys to a smooth pregnancy;

not many people know that with meditation you calm your mind, making it easier to handle the mood swings and other hormonal changes. Yoga helps strengthen the body, making it easier for you during pregnancy, labour and even after delivery.

Start with any exercise routine at a slow pace and maintain this level as at this point no one is training to be an Olympic athlete. All activities need to be under the supervision of a trained expert in that field as it is dangerous for you and the baby at this time. No activity should have any obstruction for the stomach, no pressure and no jumping.

I always advise all mothers who come for prenatal yoga to walk, as this is the safest and one of the most effective means of working out. This can be done every day which will be very beneficial for breathing as well as other issues women face during pregnancy like varicose veins, stamina, swelling and so on.

Swimming is also a good option but only if you have a clean pool in your vicinity. When you are in the water, the pressure is taken off your legs, back and stomach, making it easier for you to stretch and get an overall body workout. Swimming also cools down your body during pregnancy. But that doesn't mean you can sit in the pool the entire day. You still need to hydrate your body as you are still sweating in water but do not notice it. The body is draining itself out, therefore, always drink plenty of water when swimming.

Prenatal yoga is an activity which all soon-to-be moms should do. Yoga is an overall body workout, taking care of each and every muscle in your body, strengthening, flexing and even toning it. Yoga asanas are done differently in every step of your pregnancy, taking care of all the symptoms, side effects and mood swings. Pranayama plays a very important role during pregnancy, making your mind more conscious, stabilizing your moods, managing pain, depression, and handling irritability much better, as well as taking care of a very important symptom most women suffer from which can be dangerous, called PMS (premenstrual syndrome).

Yoga for the Third Trimester

Before beginning, prepare in the following manner:

The place: Choose a place which has fresh air and is well circulated, preferably a garden, a terrace, or a workout place in your house. Have someone present with you in the room.

The requirements: A yoga mat, a bottle of water, a hand or face towel. You can play some slow music in the background if you like.

To start: Spread the mat on the floor and sit in a comfortable position. Take 5 to 10 long breaths to relax yourself. Stretch your hands and legs to loosen the muscles. Perform the warm-up exercises mentioned in Chapter 1, p. 14, without putting any undue stress on your body.

Virabhadrasana

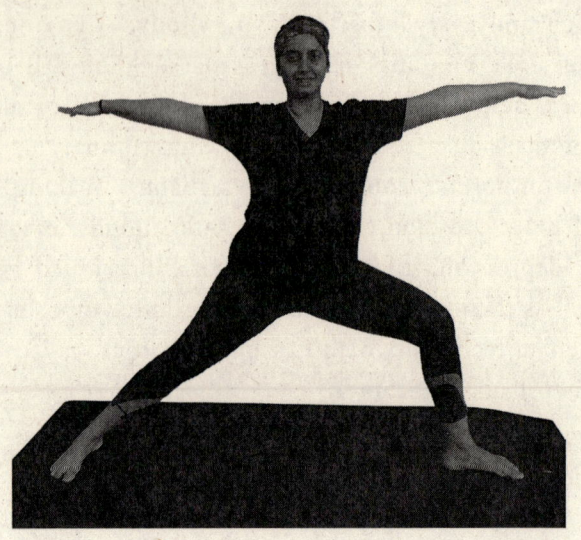

Stand straight and with an exhalation of breath, place your feet 3½ to 4 feet apart. Raise your arms parallel to the floor and open them out. Keep the right knee bent and the right thigh parallel to the floor. Stay for 30 seconds to 1 minute. Inhale to come up. Repeat the same with the other leg.

Benefits: This pose strengthens, stretches, and is even a bit of a balancing pose, that can inspire confidence and power. It strengthens the muscles of the legs, arms, shoulders, and back while stretching the calves.

Calf Stretch

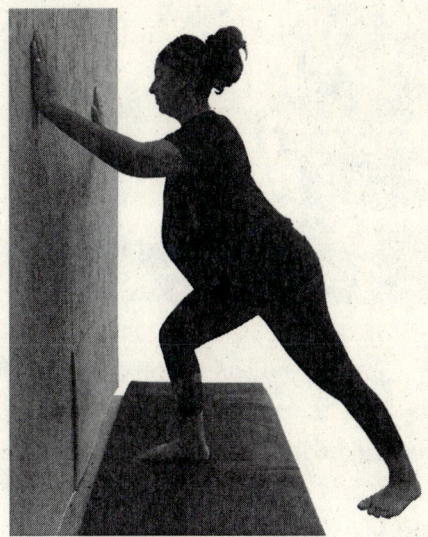

Stand to face any wall, hands raised at the front, elbows bent. Place your palms on the walls at shoulder height and lean your body weight towards the wall. Now take your right leg forward and bend a little at the knee, trying to reach the left leg, heel on the floor (make sure you do not lift the heel). Now slowly keep moving the right knee forward till you get a good stretch in the left calf, breathing normally. Hold it there for 10 counts and repeat with the other leg.

Benefits: It improves blood circulation to the calves and helps to reduce pain and swelling in the calves during pregnancy.

Back Easier

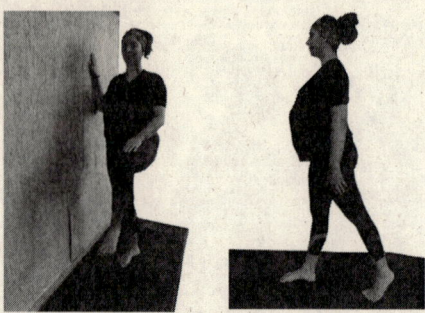

Stand beside a wall, shoulders facing the wall with a hand-distance gap. Take the support of the wall with your left hand. Lift your right leg upwards as much as you can and hold for 3 counts and slowly move your leg. Now move your leg backwards, keeping your right hand on your thigh for comfort and hold for 3 counts. Come back to the start and relax. Repeat this 5–6 times, breathing normally.

    Benefits: This pose strengthens and tones the buttock/gluteus muscles and relieves lower back pain during pregnancy.

Groin Muscle Squat

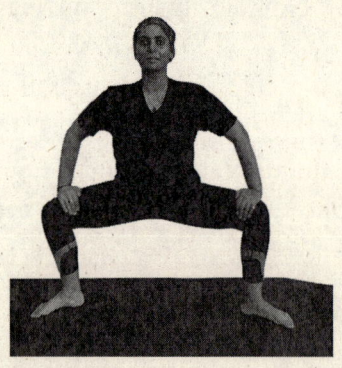

Stand with your feet a little wider than shoulder-width, toes pointing slightly outwards. Place your hands on your thighs for support and squat down, feel a good stretch across both inner thighs and hold for 3 breath cycles.

Benefits: Shortens the second stage of labour (pushing phase), shortens the depth of your birth canal and increases the pelvic diameter by more than 10 per cent.

Supported Squat

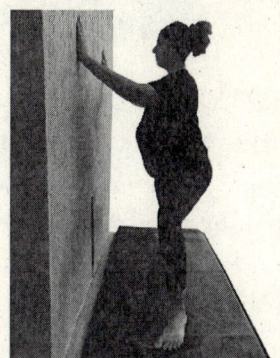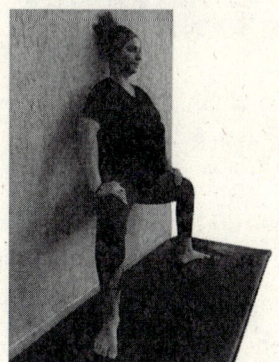

Stand to face any wall, hands raised to your sides, elbows bent. Place your palms on the walls at shoulder height. Now stand with feet a little wider than shoulder-width apart, toes pointing slightly outwards. Now slowly squat down and come up. Repeat this 5 times, keeping your breathing normal. Now turn your back against the wall for support with your hands on your thighs, squat down and hold for 3–4 breath cycles and come up. Repeat 2–3 times.

Benefits: This pose opens the pelvic region and eases out any pressure on your lower abdomen during labour.

Ankle Rotation

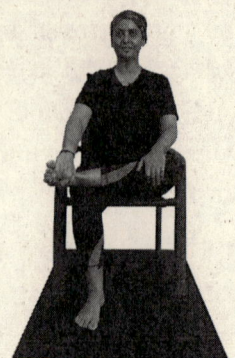
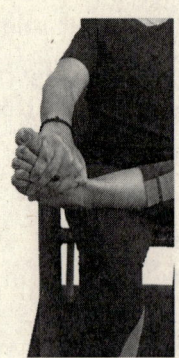

Sit on a chair, then bend the right leg up and place the foot over your left knee. Hold the right toes with the left hand. Steady the right ankle with the right hand. Rotate the right ankle around in a large circle, exploring the very perimeters of the movement. It is recommended to do 10 rotations in each direction and then another 10 with the other ankle.

Benefits: Good for stiffness and poor circulation in the feet. Helps extend the sitting time in meditation postures.

Arm Stretch

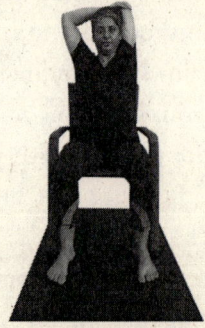
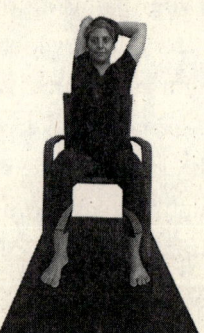

Sit on a chair with your feet apart. Raise your right hand up and behind your head and place it in the middle of your upper back. With your left hand, gently pull your right elbow back and towards your left shoulder. Hold for 3 breath cycles, and then repeat with your left arm.

Benefits: Improves circulation and flexibility in the shoulders and upper back because this stretches the arms and relieves stiffness in the shoulders.

Chest Expansion

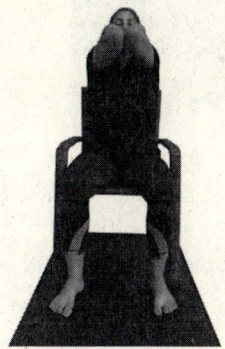 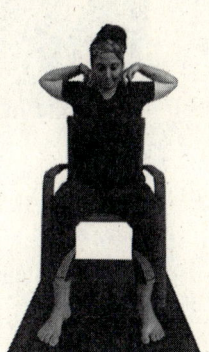

Sit on a chair with your feet apart. Now touch your shoulders with your fingertips. Bring your elbows to touch each other, pointing forward. Now move your elbows back as much as you can and slowly bring them back again, getting your elbows together. Repeat this slowly 9–10 times, breathing normally.

Benefits: This exercise releases tension from around the heart and lungs. It encourages better breathing during pregnancy.

Bhadrasana

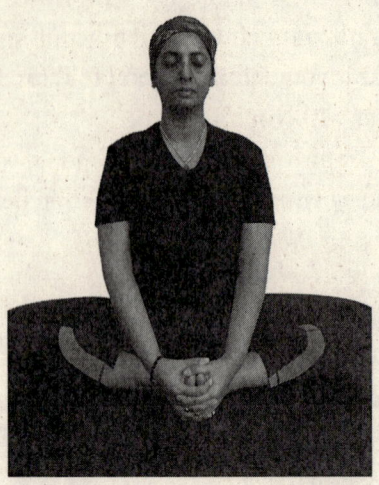

Sit in an upright position. Stretch out both legs in front of you close together. Bend your legs at the knee and bring the feet towards the body. The knees should be pointed outwards. Join the soles of the feet, with the toes and heels close together. Using the thumb, forefinger and middle finger, clasp the toes and the fore part of both the feet together. Maintain an erect posture. Widen your thighs and gently pull the knees downwards. Keep drawing the feet inwards until they are close to the perineum. Place the heels on either side of the perineum. Sit up straight. Remain in this position, breathing normally. Release the finger lock. Slowly stretch out the legs in front and return to starting posture.

Benefits: The tension from the groin muscles is relieved and tiredness from the legs removed. It also prepares you for labour.

Padmasana

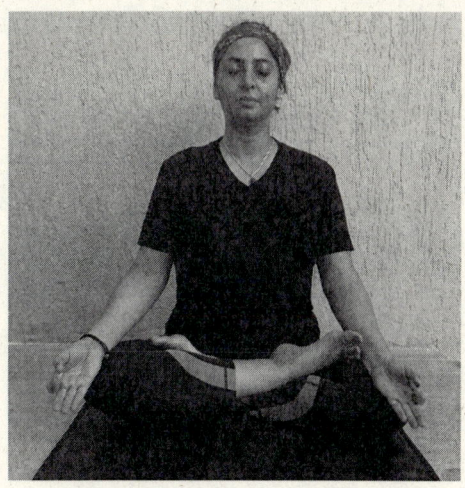

Sit with the buttocks on the floor (picture shows sitting in full Padmasana), cross the legs, placing one foot close to the inner thigh and then the other foot close to the ankle so both heels are almost at your midline. Rest the hands on the knees in Dhyana Mudra while seated in the posture. Press the hip bones down into the floor and lengthen the spine by reaching to the crown of the head. Now in this posture, do the Ashwin Mudra.

Benefits: Padmasana works on the entire body and mind. It helps in improving concentration.

Ashwin Mudra (see p. 120)

Vajrasana

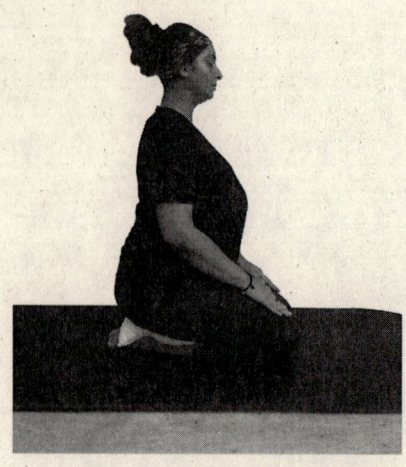

Kneel on the floor, taking the support of any object or person. Bring your toes together and separate the heels to form a V-shape, using your feet. Now place a small cushion between your buttocks and lower the buttocks on to the cushion on the back of your feet. Place your hands, palms down, on the knees. The back and head should be straight. Close the eyes, relax the arms and the whole body. Breathe normally and fix the attention on the flow of air passing in and out of the nostrils.

Benefits: Enhances digestive functions and can be practised directly after meals. Alters blood flow and nerve impulses in the pelvic regions, strengthens pelvic muscles and reduces swelling in the feet during pregnancy.

Reverse Flow

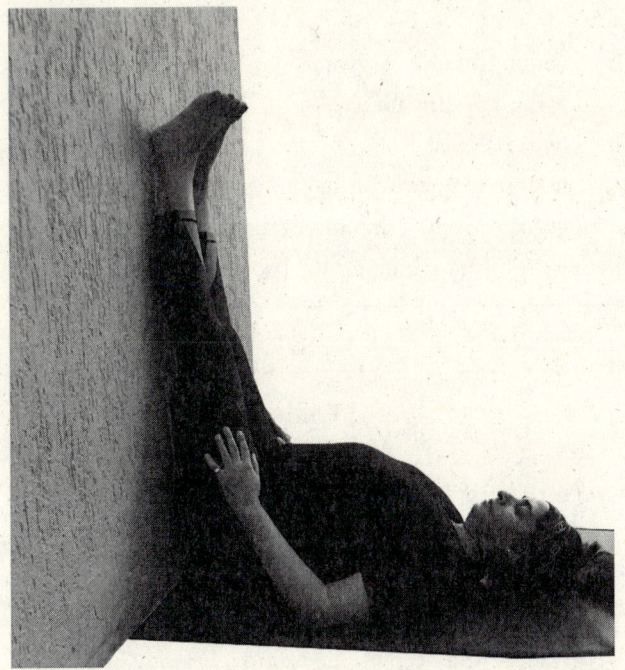

Slowly lie down on your back on the bed. Now move forward with the help of your feet on to the wall, supporting your entire body with your hands. Try getting your buttocks as close to the wall, keeping both your legs straight, with your heels and legs touching the wall. Breathing normally, stay there for 20–25 seconds and slowly come back to the starting position.

Benefits: It reduces the swelling in the legs, ankles and feet.

Myths

1. Peanuts should be avoided to prevent the baby from having a peanut allergy.
2. Give up coffee.
3. Shouldn't exercise during this time.
4. Pregnant woman shouldn't travel alone.
5. Don't buy anything for the baby before the birth.

Truth

1. Peanuts can be eaten as part of a healthy diet.
2. In small amounts, coffee is fine.
3. Nothing stops you unless your doctor says so. If you have been exercising continuously earlier then you can go ahead and keep up the routine. Just stay hydrated.
4. True, because if you go into labour, you would need someone you know beside you.
5. That would make you incompetent because you won't have time to go shopping once the baby is here.

Must Eat

1. Please consult with your doctor before making any major changes in diets or exercises.
2. It is very important to drink lot of water.
3. Avoid eating late.
4. Increase the following items in your diet, once your doctor clears them for you:
   a. Vitamin C (oranges, red bell peppers, citrus fruits, leafy vegetables)
   b. Vitamin K (bananas, beans, apricots, avocado, coconut water)
   c. Vitamin B_1 (green vegetables, fish, beans, meat, eggs, cereals, dairy products)
   d. Fibre (barley, beans, berries, Brussels sprouts)
   e. Fruits: kiwi, strawberry, melons, berries
   f. Tomatoes, beans, fibre-rich food
   g. Dal/lentils
   h. Seeds and nuts (walnuts/hazelnuts)
   i. Green leafy vegetables
   j. Porridge: oats/daliya
   k. Basmati rice
5. Food to avoid during this period:
   a. Excessive salt
   b. Chips
   c. Spicy food
   d. Too many sweets
   e. Fish with high-levels of mercury, such as shell fish, to be strictly avoided.

5

Delivery and Labour

By now you are so huge, tired and exhausted from all the preparation for the baby that it has really run you down. As the days get closer to your due date, you might feel anxious, excited and scared. Wondering what is going to happen is natural and so is feeling scared and worried about all the pain and all the scenes you saw on TV about natural births. It is important to be prepared when, even though you have discussed with your doctor that you want to go in for a normal delivery, a situation like mine might arise where a C-section is performed during delivery.

In high-pressure situations like these, it is advised to have someone you know in the room with you. You can choose whom you want there based on their ability to be your support, provide encouragement throughout the delivery and have a high tolerance level for stress.

The last few days before you're due, I suggest you spend as much time with your partner and family. If you have any older kids, spend time with them and talk to them. Helping them understand the new addition to the family and the consequent changes in the coming years will help them process the development more easily and without feeling neglected. This stands for your partners as well because your life is going to revolve around the baby once it gets here. Seeing to the feeding, changing and sleeping, might become your primary concern so it is advisable that the soon-to-be parents understand the same and support each other in whichever way possible.

By now you must have prepared for your baby's arrival by stocking up on nappies, clothes, cot, bottles and many other items. Today things have got much easier where you can have everything delivered at the click of a button from the convenience of your own home.

Many women confuse Braxton Hicks as labour contractions and run off to the hospital. The hospital usually gives you a list of things you need to get when you come in. You need to keep a hospital bag handy and ready at any given time because you are like a ticking time bomb right now. If there is anything else besides the list, do check with your hospital as they have policies that they are required to follow. I also suggest getting a feeding pillow as it is very comfortable for you as well as the baby. You can take it along with you to the hospital.

I suggest you maintain constant contact with your doctor during this time. If your doctor is travelling or not available during that time, please make sure you inquire and see to it that you are comfortable with the new doctor he has referred you to. In any case, keep a set of all medical records at hand.

What to Carry to the Hospital

1. Medical records
2. Comfortable clothes
3. Nursing bras
4. Toiletries
5. Socks
6. Baby clothes
7. Creams and lotions for your stomach and breasts
8. A set of clothes for when leaving the hospital
9. An extra set of comfortable clothes, in case you are asked to stay longer
10. Sanitary pads
11. Nightdress or top meant for breastfeeding so that it is easier for you
12. Panties; I suggest you carry a few of different brands in case you are uncomfortable with some
13. Soft and comfortable clothes for the baby
14. Innerwear for the baby like a singlet/romper
15. Socks
16. Cap that covers the baby's ears
17. Baby swaddles to wrap the baby
18. Nappies/diapers
19. Wet wipes for the baby
20. Towel for mother and one soft one for the baby
21. Baby washcloth

Signs You Are in Labour

Due to all the anxiety and sleepless nights, the arrival of your baby has been keeping you on the edge of your seat. It is important to be able to understand the various messages your body gives you. Each labour is different and you might not even experience what other women have felt. You just have to be patient and listen to your body.

The first signs of labour that I felt were abdominal cramps accompanied by low blood pressure and backache. From there, contractions start with a different frequency. You can download different apps these days that can help you keep track of these contractions and guide you along the way, making it easier for your partner. There are apps available for tracking your complete pregnancy cycle. They often come with daily tips from doctors, a chart which you can customize according to the instructions provided by your doctor and reminders for appointments or any medication. There are some apps specifically designed for tracking your contractions for frequency, duration and intensity. The contractions need to be monitored from the time you start experiencing them and need to be noted for the doctor to see. Such an app can be a godsend during this time.

From then on, your body starts doing its job and starts getting ready for the delivery of the baby. The next step is when you notice a sudden gush of fluid or even a trickle of it, which indicates your water has broken. This happens when the membranes rupture, causing amniotic fluids that were present in the uterus all this time, protecting your baby, to flow out, indicating the start of the next stage.

Thereafter, you will notice a bloody discharge like a stringy texture coming out. This is called the mucus plug; it blocks the cervix. After this, you would need to visit the loo and clear your stomach. This is a natural expulsion process where the body eliminates the stools present in the bowel and could seem as an upset stomach or diarrhoea. This is because with all the pressure you put on your pelvis during labour, the body tries to clear the system so that you do not pass stools during delivery. Sometimes women do pass stools during delivery but that is all right and nothing to be embarrassed about. This usually also depends on what you've eaten a day before you go into labour.

Before you go into labour, you might notice that you are eager to make sure everything is ready for the baby's arrival. It's called the motherly instinct. You might notice you are folding clothes or doing the dishes or taking a last-minute shower while your partner is freaking out. I would say that due to all the yoga and exercises with meditation you followed, your pain threshold is quite high compared to those who did nothing during those nine months.

Is It Time?

I suggest that the mother should be communicating with the doctor right through the contractions, even before her partner takes on the role of the mediator, so that the doctor knows where you stand on the pain threshold during your contractions.

YOU NEED TO INFORM YOUR DOCTOR WHEN

- Your water bag breaks
- You're having any symptoms like fever, severe stomach pain, diarrhoea, accompanied by dizziness, acidity, indigestion or heartburn in your lower stomach
- Bleeding
- Vomiting
- Decrease in the baby's movements
- Unbearable itching
- A feeling that something seems off

During this time of early labour, relax and rest it out as much as possible as your body needs all the rest it can get before active labour. Sit and talk to your partner. Make a list of what should be done once you deliver and return home. Watch TV and eat something nice. I am suggesting all these activities because soon it's going to be tiring and stressful for him as well. It would be nice to have a family member or friend to step in and help. You will notice you are taking deeper breaths and eating larger meals at this time. This happens when the baby has taken a position away from your chest, making it easier for you to do the above but making it more difficult to walk, sit, stand and you'd even want to pee more.

There are many labour-inducing tips that people used to follow back in the day that you might have heard about. However there is no scientific research to confirm their efficacy. These are:

- Ghee and milk
- Squatting

- Eating spicy food
- Walking
- Pineapple juice
- Rubbing your nipples to stimulate contractions

There are few yoga postures that help stimulate labour but they should be interspersed with breaks in between, if you get tired.

- Walking: 5 minutes
- Squatting: 5 minutes
- Walking: 5 minutes
- Lunges: 5 minutes
- While doing the above, keep rubbing the belly in circular motions, clockwise and anti-clockwise.
- Squat down with support as much as possible, with feet apart and toes pointing outwards. (Hold for 1 minute).
- High knees (3 to 5 minutes) holding the wall.
- Ardha Titliasana/Butterfly Pose (5 minutes, flapping legs)

Deep rhythmic breathing will help you handle contractions while letting in maximum oxygen to the mother and baby. This has to be done in counts of 10, shifting focus on one's breath as much as possible.

With sharing all this, I understand as a mother who went through this myself, that suggestions may or may not work in all cases, but if you still have the willpower to concentrate, try any of the above and try to be as calm as possible.

If you are in labour, your contractions start to become more regular and more frequent as the uterus contracts, pulls up and opens the cervix. These contractions feel like bad cramps that move down your lower back with pressure towards the front. The body prepares for the baby to come by thinning the tissue walls of the cervix, causing it to dilate. The baby is ready to come when the cervix is dilated to 10 cm, making it easy for the baby to come out.

Sometimes due to the pressure, the vaginal walls, that are thin and are also under pressure when in active delivery, tend to tear. This can be fixed but in some cases, women tend to have a long-term problem. Therefore, it is very important to exercise and take breathing and prenatal classes which play a huge role. As the baby is pushed through the canal during birth, the woman faces pressure during contractions, making it feel like wanting to pass a stool.

Many women choose to have a painkiller, Epidural, that somewhat eases the pain and tension during labour. This makes it easier and you might not feel the same intensity of pain, just pressure.

You must have heard about the term in pregnancy called Ring of Fire. This happens when the baby is about to enter the vaginal opening, stretching every part of your lower area—the vagina and the anal region. During this time, the baby's head is passing, causing it to expand. This causes an extreme burning sensation. The doctor usually takes a decision whether to make a deliberate incision on the perineum called an episiotomy. It helps prevent unwanted perineal tears which can injure the anal sphincter, and could lead to long-term issues like the loss of sensation in that area.

The baby is now delivered and is taken for suctioning and other quick tests. However, the doctor's work is still not done. He still has to deliver the placenta where the baby lived for 9 months. This is done by applying pressure again like during the delivery of your baby but is not so intense.

C-Section or Caesarean

For those who opt for a C-section or are advised a caesarean, you should know it is basically an insertion made in the lower abdomen. This process is done when there is a risk for the mother or baby and sometimes both. Doctors feel this method is the safest for mother and baby medically.

This method of delivery is painful after the painkiller wears off, making it extremely uncomfortable. The doctor suggests pain medication for this and the mother is kept in the hospital for a longer period of time. It can be very difficult for the mother who has just undergone this procedure as it usually takes 4–5 days in the hospital and even walking becomes difficult. All she is able to do for the next few days is carry her baby and feed her/him with assistance.

It is very important for you to eat a healthy diet and follow a healthy lifestyle during your pregnancy as it will help you later. You may have noticed how yoga has played such an important role in the delivery of your baby. It's never too late to start.

6

Post Delivery

On 12 September 2011, God blessed us with the most precious gift of parenthood. We welcomed our bundle of joy, who would call us Mama and Dada—magical words that we waited for so long to hear.

Once I was home, another ordeal began. Getting back in shape post-pregnancy was an uphill climb, literally. Now that you are home and healing well, you shouldn't go all out in an exercise routine, because you need to understand that your body has just gone through a drastic change in those 9 months. Looking at all those celebrities working out, getting back to their sexy figures must be driving you crazy, but listen to your body and take it slow. Start by taking your baby for strolls. I do not suggest any crash diets or strenuous workout routines.

I was 90 kg when Sayaan was born. On the table, I lost about 8 to 9 kg and the rest I had to lose on my own from then on. Usually, people start with walks in no time but I couldn't as I was suffering from something called a spinal headache. It lasted for a month. As soon as I would raise my head, my pressure would go up. I would feel giddy all the time and have headaches.

After delivery, the doctor advises you to wear a waist belt. Back in the day, they used to tie the stomach. The reasons behind this are to stabilize the organs and tighten the muscles and ligaments in the stomach area. It also strengthens the back by giving it support.

I was also dealing with becoming a new mother. All kinds of negative thoughts and doubts about my ability to become a good mother amounted to postpartum depression that many new mothers go through. Combine that with my spinal headache and the stitches due to the C-section I had undergone, I could not start any kind of workout for the next 40 days. Plus my stitches took very long to heal. It took me three months to get back to my normal self.

I assure you that you will lose the weight you put on when you were pregnant because most of it was baby weight and build-up of fluids. You will start losing weight when you start breastfeeding. You will notice that you burn down calories after you have fed your baby and you feel very hungry. It is very important that you eat healthy during this time, not only so that you don't put on weight but also because your baby is getting all the nutrients only from your milk. Your milk is formed based on the nutrients you eat during the day.

I suggest waiting for at least 6 weeks before starting any workout activity. Or take advice from your doctor and wait for his approval as each pregnancy is different. The first two weeks after delivery are the worst as your whole body is swollen and you are exhausted. Give yourself time, rest as much as you can and enjoy the time with your baby.

My experience of this period was difficult, to say the least. As I mentioned above, I was suffering from a spinal headache which lasted for 45 days. That's not the norm but a rarity. I received a lot of help to get through it but was on bed rest, advised to take a lot of fluids and even required help to start nursing my son. He would shrink from causing me any pain and refused to suckle. It took some time and various ideas to get him to start nursing properly. My husband also went through a challenging phase in the beginning. Though we didn't discuss this at that time, he came around to share his impression of the first few weeks I was home after my delivery. The sheer number of people around who were helping us—my mother, my nanny, my help, my in-laws—everyone made him feel, after a point of time, that he was not capable of taking care of this baby he had brought into the world. He even went away for a few days before he heard that my stitches had opened up and rushed back. For the first time, I saw my calm, level-headed partner start yelling at everyone that they weren't doing a good job. Pregnancy books don't talk about the father's role after the baby arrives. The world focuses on the mother and the baby, but one needs to understand that another vital person's life has changed and he is equally vulnerable at this moment. I saw this episode as an opportunity to help and support him through this phase. It is very important for both parents to work together and form a support system for the child as this helps in the long run and makes the bond stronger in this family situation.

Six weeks after the delivery, the postpartum care starts. The mother takes time to adjust to her new life with her baby. This time can be stressful and emotional as you are not getting the required amount of sleep, which disrupts your daily routine. This might also lead to depression. This is also brought about by the change in hormones that makes you susceptible to mood swings, snapping, unexplained crying, depression, irritability, sleepless nights and so on. It can get dangerous and you need to inform your doctors if you notice the following signs:

- Feeling aloof from your baby
- Feeling depressed
- Overpowered by guilt
- Not wanting to be around anyone
- Having sharp mood swings

I suggest you relax and rest as much as you can during the time your baby is napping and get help from your partner or a family member to do the changing of diapers during this time. Drink loads of water, always stay hydrated and eat healthy as this is very important for breastfeeding mothers.

There are many changes a woman goes through after delivery like:

Significant weight gain, swollen breasts, which can be very uncomfortable because your nipples will be sore as you start feeding. I suggest using a cold or warm compression on your breast during this time to soothe them. Cracked nipples are also a huge issue but can be taken care of with creams prescribed by your doctor or even breast milk.

You will notice your pelvic area is not as firm as it used to be due to all the stretching while pushing in labour, which has weakened this area. This also affects your rectal area, causing haemorrhoids to inflame and causing constipation. It is very important to have a healthy diet filled with high fibre. Your hormones are playing up and you are going to have to deal with the heat levels rising in your body, making you sweat more than you normally do.

After delivery, you will also notice a discharge. The body starts eliminating all the bad blood and toxins out. I recommend using soft non-scented pads and not using tampons during this time as this increases the risk of infections causing medical issues. Your bleeding will be minimal and not heavy. If it is heavy, contact your doctor.

Manish gifted me a treadmill as I completed 3 months of being a mother. I started my workouts and I did not miss my cardio, which lasted 30 minutes, a single day after that. I added weight training plus yoga, as time went by. I was 80 kg when I began and after eight months of good training and a balanced diet, I was close to 60 kg. So I will not say it was easy but persistence and discipline got me back to shape. Never say never because there is always a way to reach your goal. There are no shortcuts to fitness and good health.

Getting Back to Shape Post Pregnancy

Please consult your doctor before starting any exercise regime. No yoga or rigorous exercise regime should be followed until completion of 3 months after delivery. Before beginning with the workout, prepare in the following manner:

The place: Choose a place which has fresh air circulation, preferably a garden, a terrace, or a workout place in your house. You can also choose the place where your baby is sleeping or playing.

The requirements: A yoga mat, a bottle of water, a hand or face towel. You can play some slow music in the background if you like.

To start: Spread the mat on the floor and sit in a comfortable position. Take 5–10 long breaths to relax yourself. Stretch your hands and legs to loosen the muscles. Perform the warm-up exercises mentioned in Chapter 1, without putting any undue stress on your body.

POST-PREGNANCY PROGRAMME—LEVEL I

Suryanamaskars (10–15 rounds; see p. 37)

Squats (15–20 times, 3 sets)

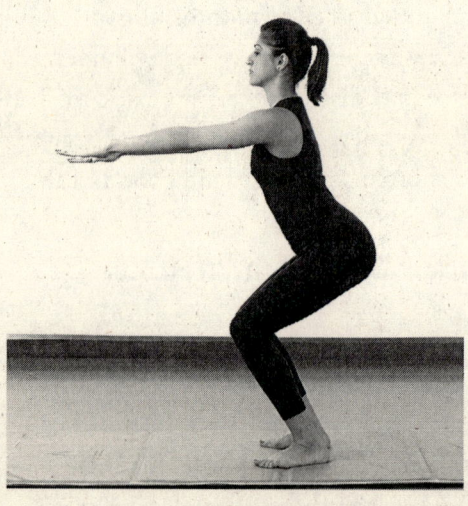

Stand straight with your hands by the side of your body. Keep your feet at shoulder-width. Now bend your knees at 90 degrees to the floor. Hold the pose and then rise back slowly.

Benefits: Squats strengthen your buttocks, abdomen and quadriceps.

Squats: Wide Legs (20–25 times, 3 sets)

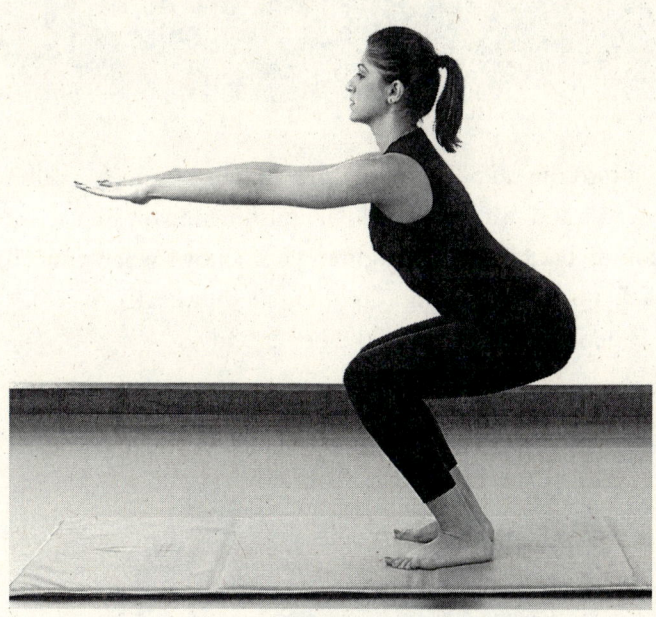

Stand straight with your hands by the side of your body. Keep your legs wide apart. Now bend at your knees, pushing your hips behind and make sure your knees do not cross your toes. Hold the pose and rise back slowly.

Push-ups: On the Knees (15–20 times, 3 sets)

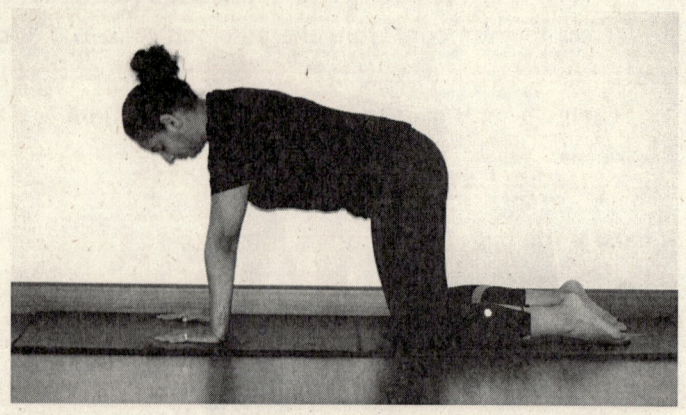

Get into the cat pose, or the Marjariasana. Bend your elbows inwards and inhale while slowly pushing down. Exhale while coming back up and straighten your elbows when you come back up. Make sure you do not arch your back.

     Benefits: Strengthens the upper body.

Upper Crunches (25–30 times, 3 sets)

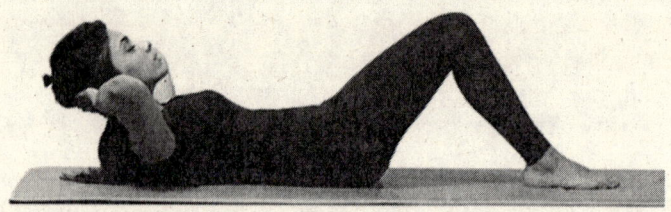

Lie on your back with your legs straight in front and hands beside your body, palms facing downwards. Slowly raise your hands behind your head and fold both your legs at the knee. Slowly keep lifting your head and crunching the upper abdominal muscles. Exhale as you come up and inhale while going down.

Benefits: Helps improve your balance by strengthening your abdominal muscles.

Leg Raises (20–30 times, 3 sets)

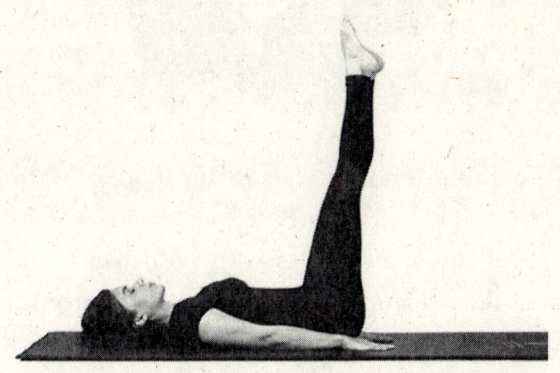

Lie in a supine position with your feet together, hands at the sides of your body and palms facing the floor. Inhale and contract your lower abdominal muscles. While exhaling, raise your feet up to a 90-degree angle from the floor. Keep moving your legs from a 90-degree to 30-degree angle, inhaling while going down and exhaling when bringing them back up, with lower abdominal contractions.

Benefits: Leg raises strengthen your core muscles.

Naukasana (hold for 15 seconds, 3 sets; see p. 54)

Dhanurasana (hold for 10 seconds, 3 sets)

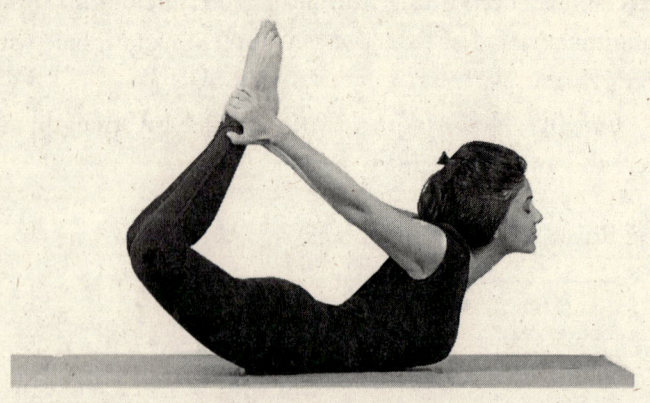

Lie in a prone position facing the floor, feet together, hands by the side and forehead on the floor. Now bend your knees, hold the ankles with both hands and, while inhaling, raise the upper body and legs up together. Hold for some time, breathing normally, and come back to the original position.

Benefits: Tones the arms, legs, stomach and back muscles.

Brahma Mudra (2 sets; see p. 59)

Kapalbhati Kriya (50–100 times; see p. 57)

Anulom Vilom (3–4 times; see p. 60)

Shavasana (5 minutes; see p. 25)

POST-PREGNANCY PROGRAMME: LEVEL 2

Suryanamaskars (25–30 rounds; see p. 37)

Jumping Jacks (30 seconds, 2 sets)

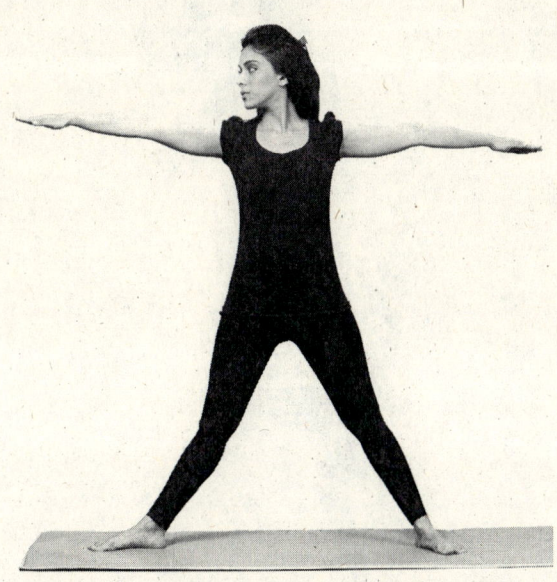

Stand straight normally. Now jump forward with your feet apart at about a distance of one foot. Then jump back to the normal position. Keep breathing normally.

Benefits: It improves blood circulation and increases the heart rate.

Squats with Front Kick (20–30 times, 2 sets)

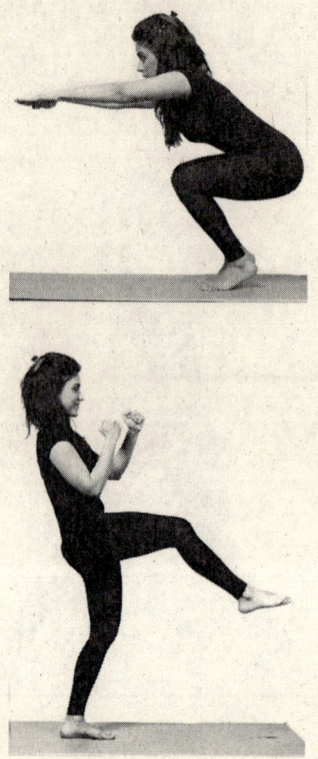

Stand straight with your feet together and your hands by the sides of your body. Keep your feet at shoulder-width. Now bend your knees at 90 degrees to the floor. Slowly raise your heels while balancing your body on your toes. Now slowly come up, raise your right leg and kick forward as high as you can while exhaling. Now go back into the squat position and slowly come back and kick with your left leg.

Benefits: Gets your heart rate up and burns more calories.

Sidekicks (30–50 times, 2 sets)

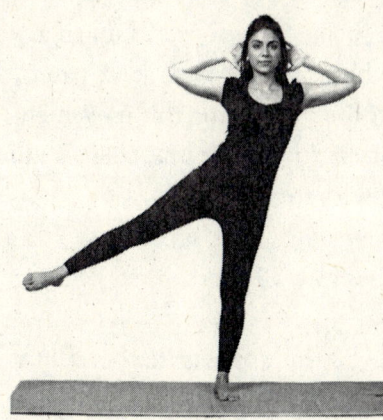

Stand with your hands behind your ears. Lift your right leg sideways as much as you can and slowly bring it down. Now repeat this, taking your leg up again and bringing it down slowly. Breathe normally and repeat this 10 times. Do this with the other leg. Come back to the start and relax.

Benefits: Strengthens and provides stability to the hips.

Push-ups: Shoulder Forward (20–25 times, 2 sets)

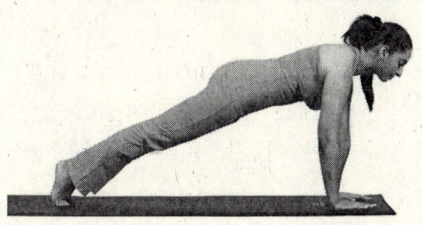

Sit in the cat pose on the floor and take both your legs behind, making sure your hands are aligned below your shoulder. The shoulders, back and hips should be in one straight line. Breathe normally when you're in this posture. While inhaling, bend your elbows as much as you can in this position and while exhaling push your palms, keeping your elbows straight. Keep repeating this movement.

Benefits: Strengthens the arms, chest, abdomen and legs, making the muscles strong.

Upper Crunches (30–50 times, 3 sets; see Level 1)

Leg Raises (30–50 times, 3 sets; see Level 1)

Naukasana (15–20 seconds, 2 sets; see Level 1)

Plank Position (15–20 seconds, 2 sets)

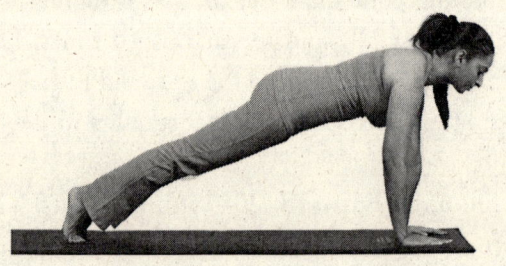

Exhale while in the cat position and put your right leg behind with the other leg. Make sure your hands are under the shoulders. The shoulders, back, hips should be in one line, parallel to the floor and once in posture, breath normally. Hold this pose for as long as you can.

Benefits: Strengthens your core.

Dhanurasana (10–15 seconds, 2 sets; see p. 170)

Brahma Mudra (10–15 seconds, 2 sets; see p. 59)

Kapalbhati Kriya (150–200 times; see p. 57)

Ujjayi Pranayam (5–10 times; see p. 61)

Shavasana (2 minutes; see p. 25)

POST-PREGNANCY PROGRAMME: LEVEL 3

Suryanamaskars (25–30 rounds; see p. 37)

Spot Running (30 seconds–1 minute, 2 sets)

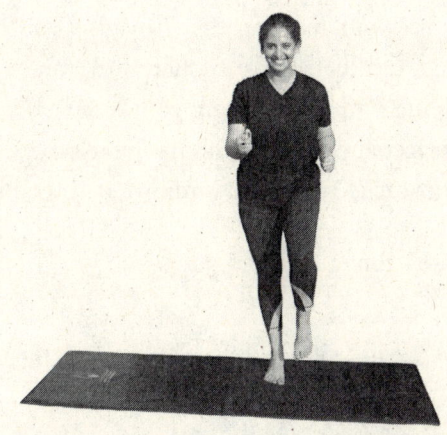

Stand straight, raise your hand and close your fist. Lift your feet one after the other, as if running, without moving from your spot. Get into a rhythmic motion and keep exhaling. Stop when you feel exhausted.

Benefits: Increases heart rate and burns calories.

Skipping (30 seconds–1 minute, 2 sets)

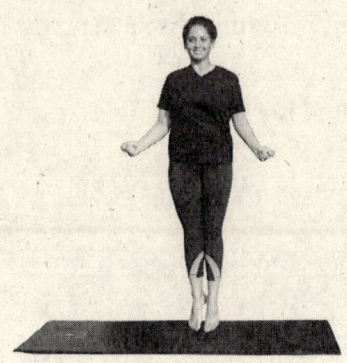

Stand straight with your feet together. Imagine you have a rope in your hand and then make circular movements at the wrist. Start jumping without bending your knees. Be soft as you land on your feet and get a rhythm going. Keep exhaling.

Benefits: It's an excellent form of cardio-vascular endurance.

Frog Jump (20–25 times, 2 sets)

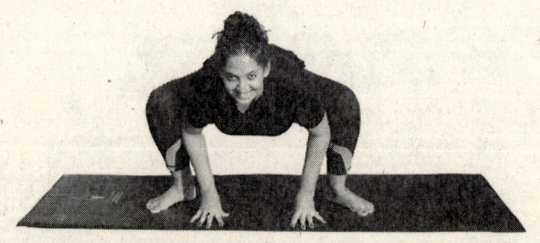

Stand straight with your hands by the sides of your body. Squat down with your knees and toes facing outwards. Move down, then jump up with the hands moving upwards. Move your body up and down like this and keep breathing in a rhythmic motion. Relax and come back to the original position.

Benefits: It helps increase heart rate and in turn helps in fat loss.

Kapalbhati Kriya: Standing (100 times, 2 sets)

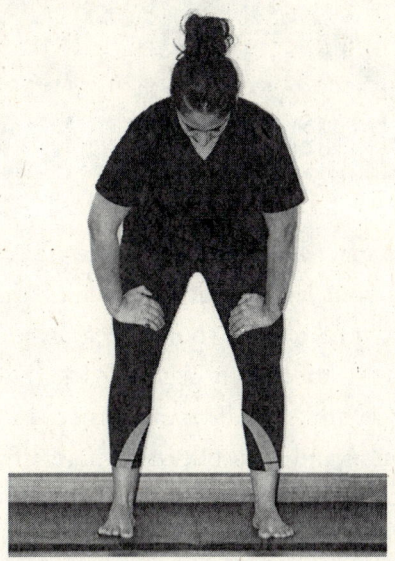

Stand straight with both hands by the sides of your body. Now slowly bend your knees, put your palms on your thighs and breathe normally for some time. Then in a quick motion, contract your abdominal muscles and forcefully exhale all the air from your lungs. Allow your lungs to fill without any effort. Once done, return back to the original position.

Benefits: Increases concentration, improves digestion, increases heart rate and blood circulation. It also stimulates and regulates the glands and reduces stress and anxiety.

Mount Climbing (30 seconds, 2 sets)

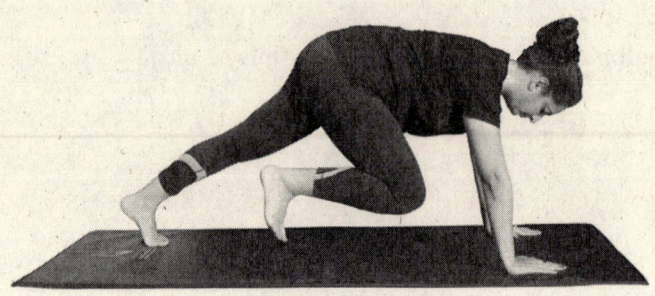

Assume Vajrasana. Move your hands forward and come on all fours. Extend your legs behind and assume the Santolasana pose. Now from here move your left leg towards your chest, bending it at the knee, then place it back. Then taking the right leg, repeat the same. Repeat this set in a continuous rhythmic motion and keep breathing normally. Once done, return to the original position.

Benefits: Improves cardiovascular endurance and strength.

Push-ups (20 rounds; see Level 2)

Upper Crunches (50 times, 3 sets; see Level 1)

Leg Raises (25–30, 3 sets; see Level 1)

Both Legs Circle (25 clockwise and 25 anticlockwise, 2 sets)

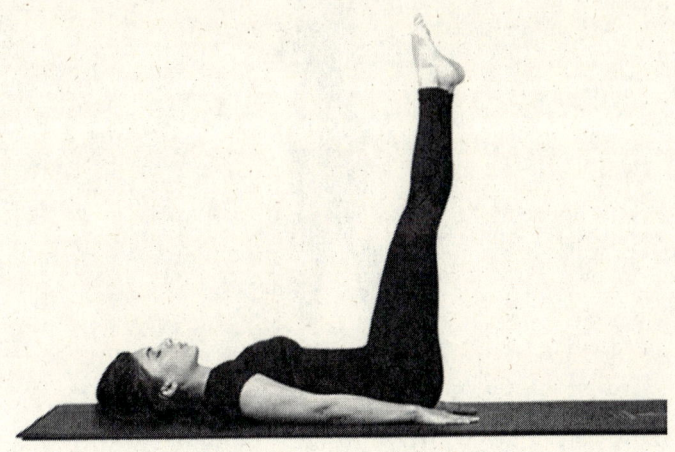

Lie in a supine position with your feet together, hands at the sides of your body and palms facing downwards. Inhale and contract your lower abdomen muscles. While exhaling raise both your legs up to a 90-degree angle from the floor. Now, keeping your legs joined, move your legs in a circular motion from right to left. Repeat the same circular motion from left to right. Inhale as you go down and exhale as you move upwards in the circle.

Benefits: This aids digestion, strengthens the abdominal muscles, burns fat in the thighs, hips and abdomen.

Kati Chakrasana (2 sets)

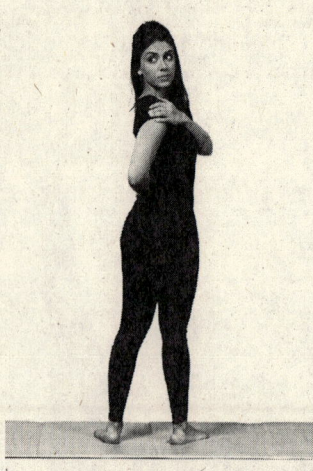

Stand straight with your feet shoulder-width apart, keeping your hands at the sides of your body. Now take your right hand behind on your lower back and keep your left hand on your right shoulder. Now twist your back towards the right side by pushing your right shoulder with your left hand, twisting as much as you can. Once in the final position, breathe normally. Do the same with the other side.

Benefits: Helps in reducing acidity, low blood pressure, and lumbar pain.

Boat Pose: On the Stomach (10 seconds, 3 sets)

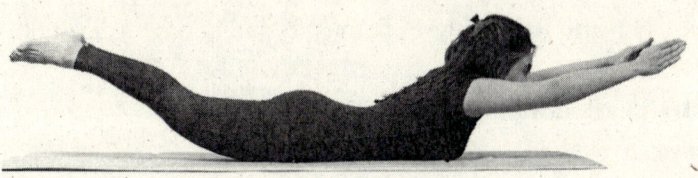

Lie down on your stomach with the feet together, hands by the sides of the body, palms resting on the floor. Slowly bring both your hands parallel to your ears, making sure that the feet are together and the toes facing outwards. Now, slowly inhale and raise your upper and lower body together at the same time, making sure the arms keep touching the ears at all times. Once your body is in this boat-like posture, hold it there and breathe normally. Slowly come back to the starting position.

Benefits: Tones and strengthens the abdominal muscles.

Makrasana (30 seconds, 3 sets)

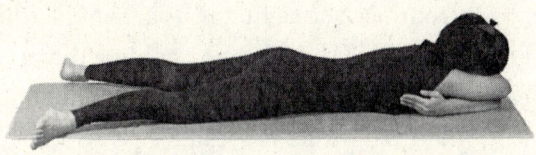

Lie in a prone position, feet together, hands by the side, palms facing upwards and forehead touching the floor. Now spread

the legs apart and turn the toes sideways, then stretch the
hands forward. Place the right hand under the left armpit,
and left hand on the right shoulder, making sure one elbow
is under the other. Relax in this position, breathing normally.

Benefits: Relaxes the back muscles and improves digestion.

Brahma Mudra (30 seconds, 3 sets; see p. 59)

Bhastrika Pranayam

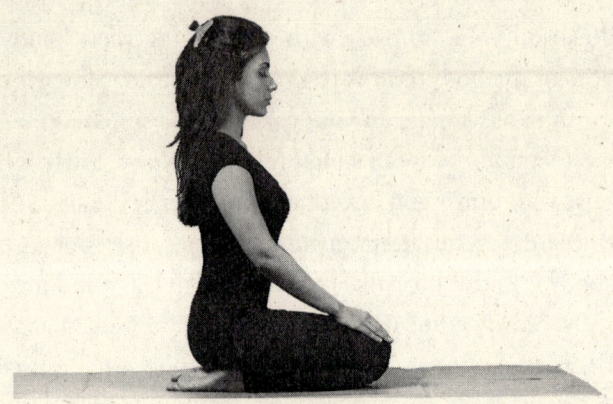

Sit on the floor in a meditative pose or in any comfortable
position. Keep your back straight and your shoulder muscles
relaxed. Do Kapalbhati Kriya 25 times, holding the last stroke
while breathing out. Then do 1 set of Anulom Vilom. This
forms one round of Bhastrika Pranayam.

Benefits: Releases toxins from the body and supplies
more oxygen to the bloodstream.

Om Chanting (5–10 times)

Tone Your Core

Warm up (see p. 14)

STANDING POSITIONS

Front Kicks (25–50 times, each leg; see Level 2)

Uddiyan Bandha (10–15 times)

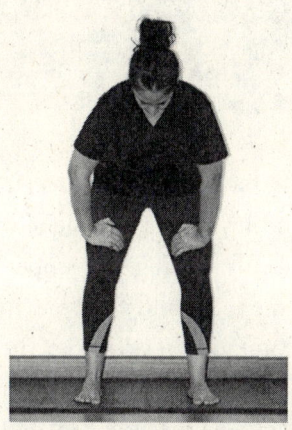

Stand straight with your feet shoulder-width apart, keeping your hands at the sides of your body. Now bend your knees, keeping your palms on your respective knees and your elbows slightly bent. Now inhale deeply and exhale forcefully, emptying your stomach and lungs. Now hold your breath out and raise your diaphragm upwards, which will make a negative pressure on your stomach. Hold this as long as you can then, while inhaling slowly, come back to the normal position.

Benefits: Better breathing capacity, reduction in chronic constipation, toning of muscles.

Trikonasana (hold for 15–20 seconds 2 times; see p. 47)

SUPINE POSITIONS

Ardha Naukasana (hold for 15–20 seconds on each leg)

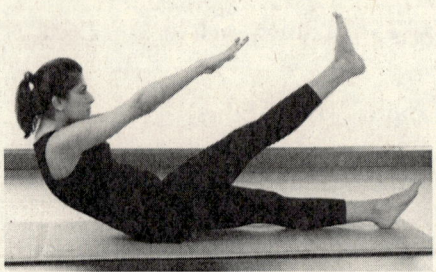

Lie down on your back with your feet together and your palms resting on your thighs. Inhale slowly and raise one leg up, simultaneously raising the upper body and hands upwards, towards the toe. Hold for some time while breathing normally. Then come down slowly to the original position and repeat with the other leg.

Benefits: Strengthens the abdominal muscles.

Ardha Triyak Naukasana (hold for 15–20 seconds on each leg)

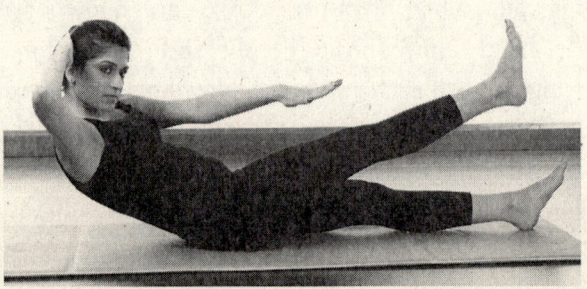

Lie on your back with the feet together and palms resting on your thighs. Inhale first and while exhaling slowly, raise your right leg up as well as your upper body while twisting your upper body to the right side. Now place your right hand behind your head. Hold for some time, breathing normally. Come down slowly to the original position and do the same with the other leg.

Benefits: Strengthens the obliques and abdominal muscles.

Setubandhasana (hold for 15–20 seconds, 2 times; see p. 53)

Naukasana (hold for 15–20 seconds, 2 times; see p. 54)

Purna Triyak Naukasana (hold for 15–20 seconds on each side)

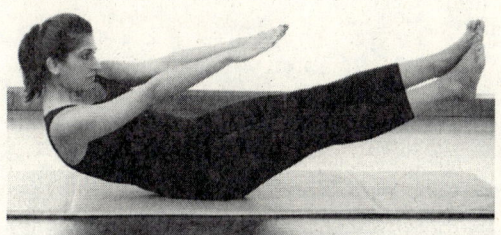

Lie on your back with your feet together and your palms resting on your thighs. Inhale slowly and raise both legs up. Then raise the upper body and hands upwards towards your toes. Now turn your full body towards the right side of your right hip. Hold for some time and come back to the original position. Repeat the same with the other side.

Benefits: Strengthens and tones the sides of the body and the abdominal muscles.

Santolasana (hold for 20–30 seconds, 2 times; see p. 40)

Santolasana Variation 2: With One Hand Upwards
(hold for 20–30 seconds on each side)

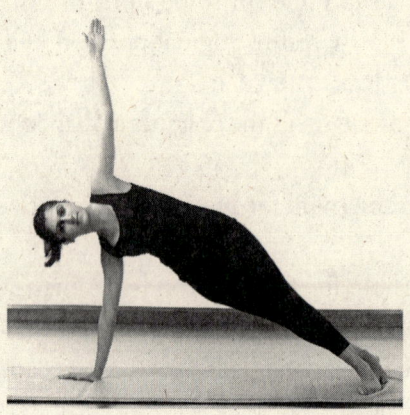

Sit in the cat pose, straighten your knees, move the shoulders forward and the buttocks downwards until the body is parallel to the floor. Turn your full body to the right side slowly and raise your left hand up to shoulder level. Make sure your upper body weight is on your right hand and lower body weight on both legs. Then come back to the original position. Repeat the same with the other side. Hold for some time, breathing normally.

Benefits: Strengthens the upper body.

Santolasana Variation 3: With Hand Behind the Back
(hold for 20–30 seconds on each side)

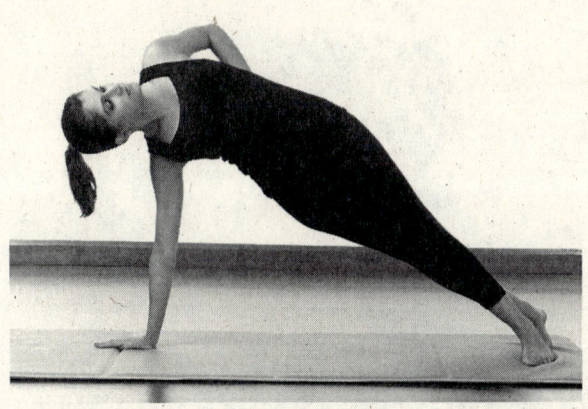

Sit in the cat pose, straighten your knees, move the shoulders forward and the buttocks downwards until the body is straight like in position No. 5 of Suryanamaskar. Now turn the body to the right side and balance it on one hand, taking the other hand behind the back and pushing the shoulder towards the ceiling. Hold for some time while breathing normally. Then slowly repeat with the other side.

Benefits: Reduces fat from the outer thighs.

Pawanmukthasana (hold for 15–20 seconds, 2 times; see p. 22)

Upper Crunches (25–50 times, 2 sets; see Level 1)

Chakrasana (hold for 10–15 seconds; avoid if you cannot do it)

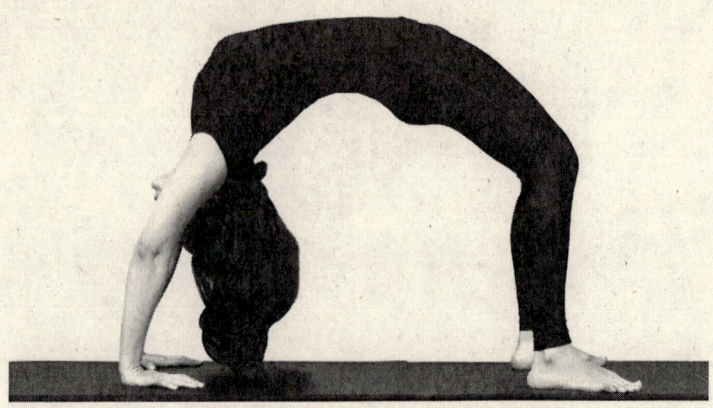

Lie in a supine position, legs together, hands by the sides, palms facing the floor. Now bend your legs at the knees, and place your feet apart on the floor close to the buttocks. Place your hands under the shoulder, palms facing down, and elbows upwards. Slowly lift the waist and upper body upwards with the help of the hands, while keeping the neck muscles relaxed. Hold this for some time, breathing normally. While coming back, first bend the elbows, put your head on the floor, then shoulder, upper back, mid-back, lower back, and finally place your buttocks on the floor and come back to the original position.

Benefits: Strengthens the abdominal and calf muscles along the biceps and improves digestion and flexibility.

SITTING POSITIONS

Ek Pada Utthan Paschimottasana (hold for 10–15 seconds
   on each leg)

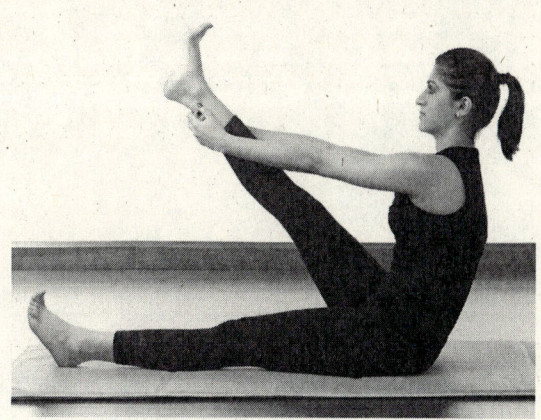

Sit on the floor with the legs straight in the front, hands by
the side of the body, and palms resting on the floor. Now
bend the right knee and hold the right ankle with both hands,
keeping the right knee straight while raising it up as much as
you can. Keep your back straight and hold it there, breathing
normally. Now slowly come back to the normal position and
repeat the process with the other leg.

Benefits: Strengthens legs and arm muscles.

Vakrasana (hold for 10–15 seconds, 2 times; see p. 50)

Ushtrasana (hold for 10–15 seconds, 2 times; see p. 20)

Paschimottanasana (hold for 10–15 seconds, 2 times; see p. 21)

Ardh Kapotasana (hold for 10–15 seconds, 2 times)

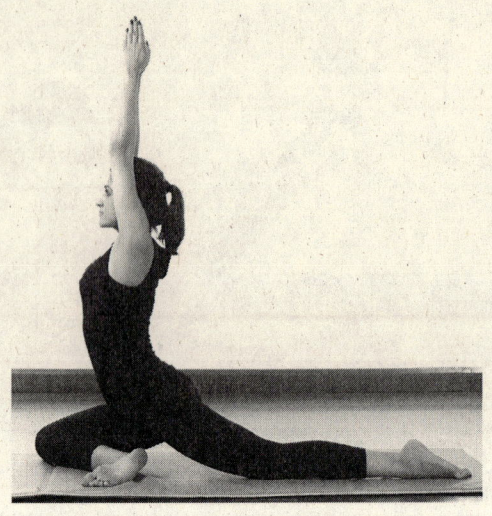

Sit on your knees in Vajrasana. Now get up on your knees, and put the right leg forward. Bend your upper body with the palms resting on the floor. Then bend your right knee, putting it on the floor, stretching the left leg behind with the knee straight and toes facing outwards. Now balance the body in the Namaskar position. Inhale and raise the hands upwards and hold for some time, breathing normally. Come back slowly to the original position. Repeat the same with the other side.

Benefits: Strengthens the hips, abdomen, arms and the back muscles.

Bhadrasana (hold for 10–15 seconds, 2 times; see p. 144)

Yog Mudra (2 times)

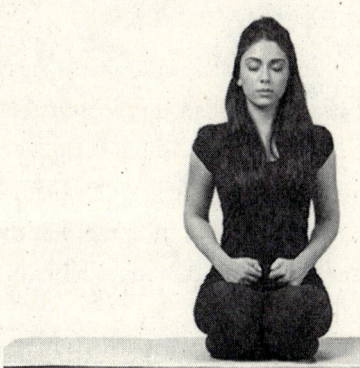

Sit in Vajrasana with your back straight and hands at the side of your body. Now close both your fists and put them on your thighs close to your navel region. Now inhale deeply. While exhaling, bend forward, touching your head on the floor and with your elbows relaxed. Hold this for some time breathing normally. While inhaling come back to the normal position.

Benefits: Improves digestive system.

PRONE POSITIONS

Sarpasana (hold for 10–15 seconds, 2 times ; see p. 41)

Dhanurasana (hold for 10–15 seconds, 2 times; see p. 170)

Naukasana (hold for 10–15 seconds, 2 times; see p. 54)

Makrasana (hold for 2–3 minutes; see p. 181)

Shavasana (hold for 2–3 minutes; see p. 25)

Grandma's Tips

1. Post-delivery, drink boiled water with ajwain. It could be made in the morning and had throughout the day. Do not keep for the next day. This helps in removing the bloating in the body. It helps in relieving constipation during and after delivery, making the strain less during passing stools. It not only cleans the stomach but in turn cleans the uterus of impurities.

    Roast 2 teaspoons of ajwain on a low flame until its fragrance starts to spread. Put this in water and bring the water to boil till it becomes brown. Let the water come to room temperature. Strain it before using.

2. For production of milk and breastfeeding it is best to eat the following:
    a. Methi ki bhaji
    b. Dill (sua) ki bhaji
    c. Chawli patta bhaji
    d. Suka narayal
    e. Halwa of rawa flax seeds and gudd (jaggery)
    f. Bhakri/bajra ki roti

3. Cover ears with cotton at all times so that no excess air enters the body as that could aggravate the bloating, though there is no scientific research on the same. It is also advised to wear a cotton pad even if you don't have your period.

4. Tie a belt or a 9-metre sari around the woman's stomach (if a normal delivery has been performed, do this after 7 days; and if it's C-section then once the stitches are removed and healed).

5. A special steam should be given to the body after delivery: Lasoon/garlic leaves + ajwain+ dhoop (camphor) + coal. Burn the coal and add the above in a vessel while standing above it without any clothes or undergarments with legs apart, letting the steam enter from below. This helps in cleansing the body and removing toxins trapped within.

6. Do not carry any weight after the delivery as the body is very weak. By doing so you would injure yourself which would affect you later in life.

7. Avoid leaving the house or travelling for 40 days after delivery as the body needs to heal and the body is very weak during this time.

8. Eat methi ladoos post-delivery. Keep them in an airtight container and have one ladoo every morning or evening with warm milk. This prevents pain in joints and back, and cold.

9. Don't forget our traditional 'maalish wali' (masseuse). Please take those massages to ease aches and pains in the body and to relax the muscles.

Breastfeeding

Myths

1. The more you eat, the more milk you produce.
2. Mothers feel they aren't making enough milk for the child.
3. The more fluids you drink the more milk you produce.
4. Women feel they should remain confined when they are breastfeeding.
5. Breastfeeding is painful.

Truth

1. It is not about the quantity you eat, it's all about the nutrition that you benefit from. Beetroot, carrots, green vegetables are recommended.
2. False. Mothers produce enough milk for their babies, sometimes in excess. It all depends on how the baby latches on.
3. Not true. Again, it's all about the nutrition a mother receives from what she eats.
4. Breastfeeding can be done anywhere and at any time. Many celebrities are spreading awareness on breastfeeding today. There are changing rooms specifically provided for babies at malls and airports.
5. Initial discomfort in breastfeeding is normal but if it extends for a long time, consult your doctor.

A Note on the Author

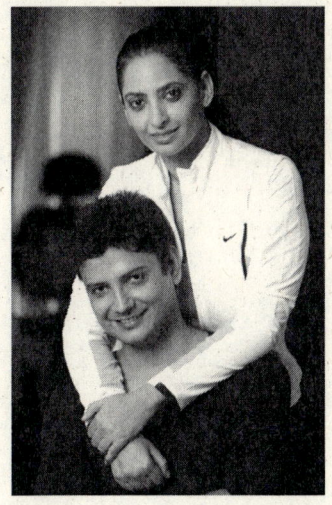

Payal Gidwani Tiwari is one of the most famous fitness and yoga experts in Bollywood and the author of *Body Goddess: The Complete Guide on Yoga for Women* and *From XL to XS* (which sold more than 75,000 copies across the country). She answered a spiritual call by turning to yoga and soon became one of its leading experts, helping a clientele which includes Sridevi, Boney Kapoor, Kareena Kapoor, Saif Ali Khan and Rani Mukerji. Payal was appointed as the fitness expert for Pond's Femina Miss India 2013 to train and guide the finalists in achieving the perfect body through yoga and distinguished fitness regimes. Payal won the Most Popular Book Award for *Body Goddess* at the Raymond Crossword Book Awards 2016–17.